Understanding Hormones for Men

Simple Steps to Avoid Complications, Reduce Medical Expenses, Decrease Stress and Live a Healthy & Proactive Life

Dr. Ashley Sullivan, PharmD

Copyright © [2024] by [Dr. Ashley Sullivan PharmD]

All rights reserved.

No portion of this book may be reproduced in any form without written permission from the publisher or author, except as permitted by U.S. copyright law.

Contents

Introduction		1
1.	Hormones Unmasked: The Invisible Forces Shaping Men's Health	3
2.	Unraveling the Mystery: Detecting Hormonal Imbalances	19
3.	The Lifestyle Labyrinth and Hormonal Harmony	27
4.	Food, the Fuel of Manhood	39
5.	Harnessing Nature's Pharmacy for Hormone Balance	59
Unlock the Power of Hormonal Health		73
6.	Navigating the Waves of Change: Understanding Age-Related Hormonal Shifts	77
7.	Navigating the Seas of Change: Understanding Andropause	85
8.	Decoding Hormone Test Results: Your Personal Guide	95
9.	Weighing the Pros and Cons of Hormone Replacement Therapy	103
10.	Planning for Long-term Hormonal Balance	117
11.	Medications Used for Hormone Balance	129

Conclusion	137
Help Others Understand Their Hormones: Leave a Review!	139
References	141

Introduction

Time keeps marching on, and we keep getting older. It's happening right now, and it's happening to everyone. With increased age comes perspective and wisdom, affording us more opportunities to share wonderful moments with the people around us. At the same time, our bodies' messages seem to get a little louder. We attribute a lot of these changes to aging, often humorously—we move a little slower, the keys become misplaced a little more frequently, and things don't operate as smoothly as they used to in the bedroom. It feels as though something may be wrong, but these topics can be a bit scary, and it can be difficult to have a serious conversation about some of our challenges.

During my years in healthcare as a pharmacist and health coach, I have seen these many times. In our youth, we often feel invincible; some of these changes are new to us, even frightening. One of the most rewarding aspects of helping people manage their health is witnessing that moment when someone realizes there are explanations for what they are experiencing. That they can learn more about these changes in their bodies and take an active approach to resolving them and improving their overall health.

Many of the processes we experience are a natural part of aging, but there is also a potential for imbalance. Like many men in their thirties, forties, or fifties, hormonal balance may be something you haven't given much previous thought to. However, it's worth paying attention to because low testosterone levels can contribute to many of the changes you may be experiencing, including low energy, mood swings, a loss of interest in sex or erectile dysfunction, hair loss, and memory problems. Low testosterone can also affect your metabolism, changing how your body processes and stores fat and maintains muscle mass.

Take John, for example, a forty-five-year-old executive who was experiencing persistent fatigue, mood swings, and a decline in his libido. Concerned about his symptoms, he sought medical advice and discovered he had low testosterone levels. Through hormone replacement therapy, John regained his energy, improved his mood, and revitalized his sex drive. His experience mirrors that of many men who find relief and restoration through addressing hormonal imbalances.

You are not alone in experiencing these changes. Even some familiar faces like Sylvester Stallone have spoken out about navigating the hormonal changes that come with aging and their personal experiences with hormone replacement therapy. You may have more in common with Rambo or Rocky Balboa than you think.

If you have spent time researching the topic, you likely have come across a wealth of information discussing various solutions to manage low testosterone, and you may have even tried a few. It can be easy to feel lost when so much information is available, but none of it seems to address the root of the problem. Much like you can't build a house without a foundation, understanding the processes taking place in your body requires looking at the big picture. What processes are occurring, and why? What changes are they causing, and how does this affect how you feel? We need to take a deeper dive and talk about the details. So, what is happening in your body, and what can you do to improve your overall health?

Chapter One

Hormones Unmasked: The Invisible Forces Shaping Men's Health

> "*A pure heart and mind only takes you so far—sooner or later the hormones have their say, too.*"
> - Jim Butcher, American Novelist

Let's start by looking at hormones in general: what are they, what do they do, and why is balance so important? Hormones are used to send messages throughout the body. They help our organs and tissues communicate with each other and with our central nervous system. These messages help define crucial functions within our bodies, ranging from sexual health to the way we feel and even the way energy is used or stored. When you feel anxious or sad, hormones can play a role in defining your emotions. When your body needs food, hormones like ghrelin are released from your intestinal tract. These let your brain know it's time to eat, making you feel hungry.

Insulin is a good example of a hormone we are all likely to be familiar with. Insulin is produced in the pancreas, primarily regulating blood sugar levels. Insulin interacts with our bodies' organs and tissues and opens the door for glucose to travel from the bloodstream to be stored or used for energy by our cells. When the body becomes less able to produce insulin or our cells become resistant to insulin, blood sugars can rise and diabetes can develop.

Cortisol is another hormone whose effects we are all familiar with. Commonly called the stress hormone, cortisol is released by the adrenal glands with adrenaline in response to stressful scenarios. The resulting "fight or flight" response gets your heart pumping, blood pressure up, and muscles tense—in other words, you're ready to *move*. While this may keep you safe under some circumstances, in many situations in modern life, these symptoms are more directly related to physical symptoms of anxiety. Consistently higher levels of cortisol over time have been linked to anxiety, depression, headaches, heart disease, and higher rates of obesity.

Thyroid hormones are instrumental in defining our baseline metabolic rate. Thyroid levels help define the way our bodies use and store energy. Low levels result in fatigue, cold intolerance, and weight gain. Let me expand on that description of thyroid hormones and their relation to men's health: Thyroid hormones, primarily thyroxine (T4) and triiodothyronine (T3), are indeed instrumental in defining our baseline metabolic rate. These hormones are produced by the thyroid gland and play a crucial role in regulating numerous bodily functions, particularly in how our bodies use and store energy.

In men's health, they specifically affect:

1. Metabolism and Weight Management:

- As mentioned, thyroid hormones significantly influence the body's metabolic rate.
- Optimal levels help maintain a healthy weight by regulating how quickly the body burns calories.
- Low thyroid levels (hypothyroidism) can lead to weight gain and difficulty losing weight, while high levels (hyperthyroidism) can cause unexpected weight loss.

2. Energy Levels and Fatigue:

- Thyroid hormones are essential for energy production at the cellular level.
- Low levels often result in fatigue and a general feeling of sluggishness.
- Men with hypothyroidism may experience decreased stamina and endurance.

3. Temperature Regulation:

- Thyroid hormones help regulate body temperature.
- Low levels can lead to cold intolerance, where men may feel cold even in warm environments.

4. Muscle Function and Strength:

- Adequate thyroid hormone levels are necessary for proper muscle function.
- Low levels can lead to muscle weakness and aches, affecting physical performance.

5. Cardiovascular Health:

    - Thyroid hormones influence heart rate and blood pressure.
    - Imbalances can increase the risk of heart disease in men.

6. Mood and Cognitive Function:

    - Thyroid hormones affect brain function.
    - Low levels can contribute to depression, difficulty concentrating, and memory issues.

7. Sexual Function:

    - Thyroid imbalances can impact libido and sexual performance in men.
    - Hypothyroidism may lead to erectile dysfunction, in some cases.

8. Bone Health:

    - These hormones also play a role in bone metabolism.
    - Long-term thyroid imbalances can affect bone density, potentially increasing the risk of osteoporosis.

9. Hair and Skin Health:

   - Thyroid hormones influence hair growth and skin health.

   - Low levels can lead to hair thinning or loss, as well as dry, coarse skin.

10. Reproductive Health:

    - Thyroid function can affect sperm production and quality.

    - Imbalances may contribute to fertility issues in some men.

It's important for you to be aware of thyroid health and to have your thyroid function checked if you are experiencing symptoms of imbalance. Regular check-ups, a balanced diet (particularly with adequate iodine intake), stress management, and maintaining a healthy lifestyle can all contribute to optimal thyroid function. If an imbalance is detected, working with a healthcare provider to restore proper thyroid hormone levels can significantly improve overall health and quality of life for men.

So, where does testosterone fit into the picture for men's health? In a sense, *everywhere*. It's produced primarily in the testes, where it plays an important role in sexual health by influencing sperm production and libido, but testosterone balance also influences many other areas. Low testosterone is associated with changes in metabolism, resulting in reduced muscle mass and increased fat production. Testosterone also affects bone density and red blood cell production, with low levels leading to higher rates of anemia and fatigue. Mood is also impacted, with higher rates of depression among men with low testosterone.

While it can be easy to become preoccupied with the various effects of low testosterone, the potential health risks associated with elevated testosterone highlight the importance of maintaining balance. When testosterone levels are high, aggressive behavior and higher rates of cardiovascular disease are observed.

Balance is crucial, and while testosterone often takes center stage, it's also important to consider the role of several closely related hormones. It can be helpful to think of these hormones as team members working alongside testosterone to keep your body functioning at its full potential. Hormones team up for some roles and may work more independently for others, but every hormone is needed to keep things running smoothly. We've already looked at thyroid hormones, so what else is on the team?

Estrogen is often associated directly with women's health, but its effects are also needed for men. Testosterone is converted to estrogen by an enzyme called aromatase, and when estrogen isn't produced properly, men may have higher rates of osteoporosis, impaired metabolism of glucose and lipids, and impaired reproductive function. Estrogen is integral in maintaining muscle mass, bone density, and sexual function in males. Some studies suggest estrogen actually has a stronger effect on suppressing increased fat distribution than testosterone in men.

Dihydrotestosterone, or DHT, is also derived directly from testosterone. Some of the effects have been more difficult to pin down in studies utilizing circulating blood levels because much of the production and activity of DHT occurs locally in cells and tissues. DHT plays a role in prostate health, cardiovascular health, and the development

UNDERSTANDING HORMONES FOR MEN

of secondary male sexual characteristics like facial hair and voice deepening.

Dehydroepiandrosterone, or DHEA, is produced primarily in the adrenal cortex and is one of the more prominent steroid hormones in humans. DHEA acts as a precursor to both testosterone and estrogen. The effects on the body are broad, ranging from neuroprotective properties and fewer symptoms of anxiety and depression to regulation of the immune response. As we age, the levels of DHEA trend lower over time.

To sum up, here is a list of the seven essential hormones every man should know about, along with their significance in your overall health:

1. Testosterone:

- Testosterone is a primary male sex hormone.

- It's crucial for muscle mass, bone density, and body hair growth.

- It influences libido, sperm production, and overall energy levels.

- It also affects mood, cognitive function, and confidence.

2. Cortisol:
- A well-known hormone, also referred to as the "stress hormone."

- It regulates metabolism, immune response, and blood pressure.

- It helps the body respond to stress.

- Chronic elevation of cortisol can lead to weight gain, anxiety, and sleep issues.

3. Insulin:
    - This hormone regulates blood sugar levels.
    - It's crucial for energy metabolism and storage.
    - Imbalances in insulin can lead to diabetes and metabolic disorders.
    - It affects weight management and overall energy levels.

4. Thyroid hormones (T3 and T4):
    - T3 and T4 control metabolism and energy production.
    - They influence heart rate, body temperature, and weight.
    - They impact mood, cognitive function, and overall well-being.
    - Imbalances in thyroid hormones can lead to fatigue, weight changes, and mood disorders.

5. Growth Hormone (GH):
    - Growth hormone promotes growth and cell regeneration.
    - It helps maintain muscle mass and bone density.
    - It influences fat metabolism and body composition.
    - It declines with age, affecting overall vitality and recovery.

6. Estrogen:
    - Estrogen is present in small amounts in men.

- It's important for bone health and cognitive function.
- It helps regulate cholesterol levels.
- Imbalances in estrogen can affect prostate health and body fat distribution.

7. Melatonin:
   - This is the hormone that helps regulate the sleep-wake cycle (circadian rhythm).
   - It influences sleep quality and duration.
   - It acts as an antioxidant in the body.
   - It's important for overall health, mood, and cognitive function.

Understanding these hormones and maintaining their balance is crucial for men's overall health, energy levels, mental well-being, and long-term vitality. Regular check-ups, a healthy lifestyle, proper nutrition, and stress management can help maintain optimal hormonal balance.

As you can see, hormone functions play a variety of roles in men, affecting sexual function, fertility, body mass, metabolism, prostate health, bone health, heart health, mood, and cognition. So, with all of these factors (and many more) coming into play, what systems are in place that help define when and how much of these hormones are released?

The Endocrine System: The Mastermind Behind Hormone Production

If you have ever worked in a relatively large organization, you know how important (and sometimes challenging) communication can be. Getting everyone on the same page and working toward the same goals within their individual roles requires a lot of coordination. This is particularly true if everyone needs to pivot fairly quickly and adapt to changes.

In some ways, the body can be thought of similarly. Individual cells, organs, and organ systems need to be able to work together—and adapt quickly at times. To do their job well, they need a way to communicate. The endocrine system fulfills this need, providing a way for every organ in the human body to communicate.

Needs are interpreted, signals are sent, and hormones are released to pass the message along. Sometimes, hormones are produced locally; sometimes, they are produced by dedicated glands whose messaging has a broad reach. While a fairly simplistic analogy, if the body designated a CEO of the endocrine system, the hypothalamus would fill this role.

The hypothalamus sends messages to the pituitary gland, which produces messages to multiple glands and organs in the body, resulting in hormone release. These targets include the thyroid gland, adrenal glands, and testes, the primary source of testosterone.

As an example of a rapid response, when you are under stress, the hypothalamus signals the adrenal gland. Cortisol is released and acts in multiple areas of the body, promoting the activity of the sympathetic nervous system. The net effect is commonly called a "fight or flight" response—your muscles tense and your heart is pounding.

Cortisol provides a great opportunity to examine how the timing of hormone release can vary. In some situations, this release and its effects occur very quickly, but there are also waves that occur daily. For example, your baseline cortisol levels are higher in the morning to help you get up and moving, decreasing throughout the day.

Sometimes, these waves play out over a much longer time frame. In the case of testosterone, the circulating baseline levels tend to peak in a man's late teens. This is followed by a gradual decrease of about 1 percent per year beginning around age thirty. There is a potential for variation, of course, but understanding how these changes may affect you and your body can help you achieve better control of your overall well-being.

Decoding Hormonal Health: Why It Matters for Men

We've all been there. Something doesn't feel quite right, but it may be difficult to put your finger on it. Learning more about the signals your body is sending can help you start to move beyond the uncertainty of a potential problem so you can begin to address it. As part of this process, we can find answers to some important questions:

- What are some potential reasons why I feel the way I do?

- Is it a cause for concern or a sign of a deeper underlying problem?

- What can I do about it?

Assessing whether or not there is an underlying problem requires the help of your doctor. When you have had regular check-ups in the past, they may have felt formulaic—there are set questions you are always asked, and many of your answers may have been the same over time. It's important to have a sense of agency in this relationship and have questions of your own.

Hormonal changes can occur relatively slowly and include areas that may not come up in conversation as frequently, like loss of interest in sex. This, combined with a general lack of energy and weight gain, can be a sign of low testosterone levels. Keeping your doctor informed helps to ensure you are receiving the right tests and, ultimately, the right treatments.

Mood changes are important to talk about as well. For instance, if you have low testosterone, you may be more likely to feel down or depressed. Higher levels of testosterone can cause mood swings and increased aggression. Balance is key—not only for testosterone but for all hormones.

Many factors beyond age-related changes within the body influence hormonal balance. Eating a diet with a lot of processed food and added sugar can disrupt insulin balance. This can then lead to weight gain and a higher risk of developing diabetes.

Stress is a part of daily life. If you are not acknowledging your stressors and actively taking steps to manage them, it can open the door to further imbalances. Chronic stress can cause a build-up of cortisol and bring on the potential for a wide range of concerns. These include changes in eating habits (you're more likely to crave calorie-dense "comfort food" when cortisol levels are high), difficulty sleeping, and an increased risk for high blood pressure and cardiovascular disease.

We could go on and on about the research and the associated health risks of hormonal imbalances. Avoiding health concerns is certainly important, but taking steps to maintain hormonal balance also allows you to be the best version of yourself. When your testosterone levels are balanced, you are more likely to feel mentally stable, energized, and confident, including in the bedroom.

It can be all too easy to shrug off potential signs of an imbalance, so it's important to know what to watch for.

Debunking Hormonal Myths

In the realm of men's health, hormones play a crucial yet often misunderstood role. As we navigate the complex landscape of male physiology, we need to acknowledge the numerous myths and misconceptions that have taken root, potentially leading to confusion and misinformed decisions about health and wellness. Understanding the truth behind these hormonal health myths is not just about separating fact from fiction—it's about empowering men to take control of their well-being with accurate knowledge.

Hormones are the body's chemical messengers, orchestrating everything from metabolism and mood to sexual function and muscle growth. Yet, the nuances of hormonal health in men are frequently oversimplified or misrepresented in popular media and even some medical circles. This can result in delayed diagnoses, unnecessary treatments, or missed opportunities for improving quality of life.

In this debunking exercise, we'll examine six common myths about men's hormonal health. By addressing these misconceptions head-on, we aim to provide clarity and foster a more comprehensive understanding of how hormones affect men's bodies and minds. Armed with this knowledge, you can make more informed decisions about your health, engage more effectively with healthcare providers, and take proactive steps toward hormonal balance and overall wellness. Let's dive into these myths and uncover the truths that every man should know about his hormonal health.

Myth 1: "Low testosterone only affects older men."

Reality: While testosterone levels naturally decline with age, low testosterone can affect men of all ages. Factors such as stress, obesity, poor diet, and certain medical conditions can lead to low testosterone in younger men as well. It's important for men of all ages to be aware of symptoms like fatigue, decreased libido, and mood changes, which could indicate hormonal imbalances.

Myth 2: "Testosterone replacement therapy (TRT) causes prostate cancer."

Reality: There is no conclusive evidence that TRT causes prostate cancer. While testosterone can accelerate existing prostate cancer growth, properly monitored TRT in men without prostate cancer is generally considered safe. Regular prostate screenings are important for men on TRT, but the therapy itself doesn't increase the risk of developing prostate cancer.

Myth 3: "Men don't have estrogen, so it's not important for their health."

Reality: Men do produce estrogen, albeit in smaller amounts than women. Estrogen plays crucial roles in men's health, including bone density maintenance, cognitive function, and cardiovascular health. An imbalance in the testosterone-to-estrogen ratio can lead to health issues, highlighting the importance of estrogen in men's overall hormonal health.

Myth 4: "Hormone imbalances only affect physical health, not mental health."

Reality: Hormones significantly impact both physical and mental health in men. Imbalances can lead to mood swings, depression, anxiety, and cognitive issues. For instance, low testosterone has been linked to depression, while thyroid imbalances can affect mood and cognitive function. Understanding this connection is crucial for comprehensive men's health care.

Myth 5: "Once you start hormone replacement therapy, you have to continue it for life."

Reality: While some men may benefit from long-term hormone therapy, it's not always a lifelong commitment. The duration of treatment depends on individual factors, underlying causes, and response to therapy. Some men may be able to discontinue treatment after addressing lifestyle factors or underlying health issues that contributed to the hormonal imbalance.

Myth 6: "High testosterone levels always lead to aggression and road rage."

Reality: The link between testosterone and aggression is often oversimplified. While very high levels of synthetic testosterone (as in steroid abuse) can lead to increased aggression, normal to high-normal testosterone levels within physiological ranges are not directly correlated with aggressive behavior. In fact, balanced testosterone levels are associated with better mood regulation and emotional well-being.

Understanding these realities can help you make more informed decisions about your hormonal health and seek appropriate care when needed. By debunking these common myths, we've taken the first step toward a clearer understanding of your hormonal health. However, this is just the beginning of our journey into the intricate world of hormones. As we've seen, the reality of hormonal balance is far more nuanced than many of us have been led to believe. It's a complex interplay of various factors, affecting not just our physical health, but our mental and emotional well-being as well.

With this foundation of knowledge, we're now ready to delve deeper into the mysteries of hormones and learn how to spot the signs of trouble before they escalate into more serious health issues. In the next chapter, we'll explore the subtle signals your body may be sending—from unexplained fatigue and mood swings to changes in libido and body composition. We'll unravel the complex language of hormones, teaching you how to interpret these signals and when to seek professional help. By becoming more attuned to your body's hormonal cues, you'll be better equipped to maintain optimal health and address potential imbalances early on.

Chapter Two

Unraveling the Mystery: Detecting Hormonal Imbalances

> *.. Prevalence of hypogonadism has been estimated to be 39% in men aged 45 years or older presenting to primary care offices in the United States."*
> - Rivas, 2014

Spotting the Warning Signs: Symptoms of Hormonal Imbalances

Our hormones have the potential to fly under the radar. Many of the changes we experience can be written off as minor inconveniences or simply attributed to other challenges we may face. Are you feeling tired today? It's easy to chalk that up to not getting as much sleep as you'd like or to a particularly rough stretch at work.

Take a moment and step back. Getting wrapped up in the daily grind may cause you to lose sight of some longer-term patterns. Have there been larger changes in your stress level or mood over time? How about your energy? Are you eating a healthy diet and staying active but still gaining weight?

These can be more subtle patterns that are easy to miss, partially because it's so easy to find a more immediate cause to pin things on. For instance, maybe you have been managing depression for years and have become somewhat accustomed to the ups and downs. You've approached your depression directly, and medications and coping techniques help, but you still find yourself stuck in a rut at times. This is the nature of depression, but hormones like testosterone do have the potential to impact this.

Other signs of low testosterone may be easier to pin directly on potential hormonal imbalances. Take gynecomastia or breast enlargement. If you notice this happening and haven't spent extra time on the bench press, you might suspect something is up. The same could be said of erectile dysfunction, as it could be more easily linked to changes in testosterone.

It's important to keep in mind that each of these concerns has a variety of potential causes. Certain medications can cause gynecomastia. Thyroid levels impact your energy. Not all mood changes are the result of a hormonal imbalance. This highlights the importance of giving your doctor the whole picture so you can dive deeper and get to the heart of the problem. Great communication leads to great treatment.

Hormonal imbalances can present with subtle symptoms that we often overlook or attribute to other factors. It's crucial to pay attention to patterns in our energy levels, mood, weight changes, and physical symptoms. While some signs may be more evident, like gynecomastia or erectile dysfunction, others can be easily missed. By being aware of these potential warning signs and communicating openly with our healthcare providers, we can better identify and address any underlying hormonal imbalances.

Understanding the Underlying Causes: Why Do Hormonal Imbalances Occur?

Hormones can potentially disrupt important processes in our bodies and change how we feel, but how do they become imbalanced? In some ways, maintaining your health could be compared with sports or games of skill.

Take golf, for instance. Some factors are outside your control. The weather, the wind, the course you agreed to play despite the annoying amount of sand traps. You can't control everything. Some things also tend to add up or feed into one another. That light drizzle is picking up, and you are starting to feel a bit chilly; the grass is wet, and you need to adjust your shots. You brought an umbrella and a towel to keep your club handles dry, though, so that helps. You can choose which club to swing, how hard to swing it, and even try to account for that slice. In other words, you've got some tools at your disposal.

Some imbalances in your body are beyond your control without medical intervention. For example, low thyroid levels, or hypothyroidism, can sometimes be the result of your own immune system causing inflammation in the thyroid gland. In some ways, this is a bit like the weather in that it does not result from something you did or didn't do. Low thyroid levels can cause your metabolism to slow down, making you feel more sluggish and your weight more difficult to control. Medication may be needed to help replace the missing thyroid hormones.

Your lifestyle can influence other imbalances, and this is where your choices can have a solid impact in preventing problems before they arise. If you are eating a lot of processed foods, these are often very high in saturated fat, salt, and sugar content. Over time, this leads to the potential for gaining weight, developing insulin resistance, and can ultimately even lead to type 2 diabetes. Eating more whole foods, like fresh fruits and vegetables, lean meats, and whole grains, can provide plenty of healthy nutrients, as well as stabilizing your blood sugar and insulin levels.

Much like diet and exercise routines are tools at your disposal, so is your ability to manage stress. This is a learned skill that requires some honest reflection, and you'll be stronger for it. When stress is left unmanaged, the stress hormone cortisol begins to cast its far-reaching shadow. Ultimately, the balance of other hormones is also affected, including those responsible for hunger, metabolism, and even testosterone. The effect is more cravings for foods that are high-calorie and have low nutritional value, a higher risk of insulin resistance and increased weight, lower libido, and the potential for damage to reproductive organs. Take steps to manage your stress so it doesn't manage you.

In today's fast-paced world, stress has become an unwelcome companion for many men, silently wreaking havoc on hormonal balance and overall health. The intricate dance of male hormones, particularly testosterone and cortisol, can be easily disrupted by chronic stress, leading to a cascade of health issues ranging from fatigue and weight gain to decreased libido and mood disorders. Stress management has become increasingly important, so to help, we have provided a step-by-step guide on stress management, specifically tailored for men"s hormonal health. Following the steps will help prevent hormonal havoc:

1. Recognize Stress Signals:

- Identify physical symptoms (e.g., tension, fatigue, headaches).

- Notice emotional changes (irritability, anxiety, mood swings).

- Be aware of behavioral shifts (sleep disturbances, changes in appetite).

2. Prioritize Sleep:

- Aim for seven to nine hours of quality sleep nightly.

- Establish a consistent sleep schedule.

- Create a relaxing bedtime routine.

- Avoid screens for one to two hours before bed.

3. Exercise Regularly:

- Incorporate 150 minutes of moderate aerobic activity weekly.

- Include strength training two to three times a week.

- Try stress-reducing activities like yoga or tai chi.

4. Practice Mindfulness and Meditation:

- Start with five to ten minutes daily, gradually increasing.

- Use guided meditation apps if needed.

- Focus on deep breathing exercises.

5. Optimize Nutrition:

- Eat a balanced diet rich in whole foods.

- Include foods that support hormone health (e.g., fatty fish, nuts, leafy greens).

- Limit processed foods, excessive caffeine, and alcohol.

6. Manage Time Effectively:

- Prioritize tasks and set realistic goals.

- Use time management tools or apps.

- Learn to say "no" to non-essential commitments.

7. Cultivate Social Connections:

- Spend quality time with family and friends.

- Join clubs or groups aligned with your interests.

- Consider joining a men's support group.

8. Develop Healthy Coping Mechanisms:

- Engage in hobbies or creative activities.

- Practice journaling to process thoughts and emotions.

- Use humor and laughter as stress relief.

9. Limit Technology Use:

- Set boundaries for work emails and calls outside of work hours.

- Take regular breaks from social media.

- Create tech-free zones or times in your home.

10. Consider Supplements (under professional guidance):

- Explore adaptogens like ashwagandha or rhodiola.

- Consider omega-3 fatty acids for overall health.

- Discuss vitamin D supplementation with your doctor.

11. Practice Relaxation Techniques:

- Try progressive muscle relaxation.

- Use aromatherapy with calming scents like lavender.

- Explore biofeedback or float therapy.

12. Regular Health Check-ups:

- Schedule annual physicals and hormone level checks.

- Discuss any concerns with your healthcare provider.

- Monitor stress-related health markers (e.g., blood pressure, cortisol levels).

13. Set Boundaries:

- Establish clear work-life boundaries.

- Communicate your needs effectively in relationships.

- Learn to delegate tasks when possible.

14. Engage in Nature:

- Spend time outdoors regularly.

- Try forest bathing or hiking.

- Incorporate plants or natural elements in your living space.

By implementing these strategies, you can take control of your stress levels, optimize your hormone balance, and pave the way for improved physical, mental, and emotional well-being. Remember, managing stress isn't just about feeling better in the moment—it's an investment in your long-term health and vitality as a man. Be patient with yourself and focus on consistent, small improvements. Tailor these steps to fit your lifestyle and preferences, and don't hesitate to adjust your approach as needed. By effectively managing stress, you can significantly improve your hormonal balance and overall well-being.

So, while we've seen that some hormonal imbalances may be beyond our control, requiring medical intervention, others can be influenced by our lifestyle choices. By adopting a balanced diet rich in whole foods, engaging in regular exercise, and practicing effective stress management techniques, we can take proactive steps to maintain hormonal balance and overall well-being.

Taking Action: When to Seek Medical Help

Armed with the knowledge of the kinds of changes low testosterone can cause, the next step is to talk about your symptoms with your doctor. The best way to confirm whether a hormonal imbalance like low testosterone is present is to have levels checked directly. Symptoms like persistent fatigue, erectile dysfunction, mood changes, or difficulty with weight gain are reason enough to schedule an appointment. Even if your testosterone levels are normal, you may be able to determine another cause and develop a plan to start feeling like yourself again.

If you hesitate or skip your appointments and low testosterone levels are missed, there is a potential for weightier consequences over time. Low testosterone makes it harder to maintain bone density, leading to osteoporosis and an increased fracture risk. Muscle mass is harder to build and maintain. The risk of developing cardiovascular disease is increased.

The best way to make sure you stay on top of your health is to schedule regular appointments with your primary care provider. Testosterone levels start to decline as men enter their 30s and continue to drop at a rate of about 1 percent each year. When you stay consistent with your check-ups, you'll be more likely to catch any potential imbalances before they become a larger problem. Don't ignore symptoms or put off seeing your doctor. Keep those regular appointments, communicate openly about any changes you are experiencing, and have your labs checked. Being proactive and having open conversations with your healthcare provider is key to identifying and addressing hormonal imbalances early on. By taking action and seeking medical help when needed, you can take control of your health and well-being.

Chapter Three

The Lifestyle Labyrinth and Hormonal Harmony

"Stress is caused by being 'here' but wanting to be 'there.'"
- Eckhart Tolle, German writer

Stress: the Hidden Hormone Playing Havoc

In recent years, particularly while navigating the challenges of 2020 and the COVID-19 pandemic, the importance of mental health has come more into focus for many people. This heightened awareness is wonderful because mental health has a tendency to be overlooked or swept under the proverbial rug, often due to societal stigmas. Negative emotions like anxiety, sadness, anger, guilt, and fear are uncomfortable but normal experiences. It's important to acknowledge and process these feelings in a healthy way rather than ignoring or suppressing them. Our feelings, especially those perceived as negative, can be uncomfortable to talk about at times, but ignoring stress and neglecting our emotional well-being has very real consequences that can manifest in various aspects of our lives.

It's also easy to get caught up in daily routines and lose track of the here and now. Deadlines, appointments, traffic, the price of groceries, re-hashing conversations—our minds are constantly pulled into planning, annoyance with the present, or replaying things that have already happened. We may not even be aware that it has been quite some time since we've taken a moment to slow down and just be present.

Stress has an insidious tendency to build, and it is extremely pervasive in American life. Americans are 20 percentage points more likely to report feeling stressed compared with the worldwide average. Over half of Americans report feeling stressed on a daily basis. Workplace stress is particularly common, with nearly two-thirds of respondents stating they are ready to move on from their current jobs.

When stress builds, so does the hormone cortisol. In the short term, our muscles tense and our heart races. Our bodies are conditioned to keep us safe when we need to run from a bear, but these same responses also happen when we sit in traffic or prepare for a Monday morning meeting. It seems that modern life presents us with a lot of bears to run from.

In the longer term, consistently elevated cortisol levels begin to lead to hormonal imbalances. The signs this is occurring can be related to how we feel—irritable, tired, or having trouble concentrating. The signs can also be more physical, like a loss of bone density or muscle mass.

Stress management is crucial, and it needs to be intentional. Taking time for yourself isn't selfish; returning to your responsibilities while feeling more calm and centered benefits everyone. There are a number of ways to help manage stress, and a lot of it has to do with your mindset.

Getting good, consistent exercise is an excellent stress reliever in addition to keeping you physically fit. If hitting the gym isn't your thing, simply getting outside and taking a walk can be beneficial. Remember to take a moment to appreciate your surroundings, the smells, the sights, the trees, the architecture of the buildings—whatever captures your interest in the moment. Take a break from planning or worrying and let yourself enjoy it.

This idea of "living in the present" extends itself directly into mindfulness. Take some time to challenge those intrusive thoughts and focus on yourself or your immediate surroundings. This can be achieved through thought exercises, where each time you find your mind wandering into the "what-ifs," you simply turn it off and consciously regain focus on the here and now. Mindfulness can also be extended into forms of meditation, breathing exercises, or yoga. Meditation has been found to effectively decrease cortisol levels in clinical research.

A benefit of mindfulness is that its tenets can be practiced anywhere. The next time you're stuck in traffic, take a moment to breathe. You can't do anything about the car in front of you, but you can control how you respond to the situation. It is what it is, you're doing what you can, and that is enough. There may be plenty of situations where reminding yourself of this would be beneficial.

A potentially trickier aspect of stress to address is our relationship with sleep. Stress makes getting quality sleep difficult, and a lack of quality sleep leads to stress. Taking steps to break the cycle can get you closer to the seven to nine hours of sleep each night recommended by the National Sleep Foundation.

The Sleep-Deprived and the Hormonally Challenged

You toss and turn, and glancing at the clock only makes it worse. Maybe your mind just keeps running while you're trying to rest or you just can't seem to drift off to sleep the way you used to. Not getting enough sleep is common, with more than a third of adults in the United States reporting they aren't getting the recommended amount of sleep, leaving them feeling tired during the day for at least half of the week.

We all know what it feels like when we don't get a good night's rest—we are groggy, less productive, and more irritable. What might not be as readily apparent is the impact a lack of sleep can have on hormonal balance. As we sleep, our bodies use this time to repair our cells. Being deprived of this time is associated with changes in cortisol levels.

Over the course of a typical twenty-four-hour period, hormones are released according to a standard circadian rhythm. Assuming a bedtime of about 9 or 10 P.M., cortisol levels will be lowest at about midnight, or two to three hours after falling asleep. At this time, cortisol levels begin to build steadily throughout the morning and peak about twelve hours after your bedtime before steadily decreasing again throughout the day. Individuals getting restricted amounts of sleep (about four hours, for instance) have consistently higher cortisol levels. Sleeping for shorter periods of time, along with elevated cortisol, is also associated with changes in metabolism that can lead to obesity and diabetes.

Fortunately, there are some simple first steps you can take to promote more consistent, better-quality sleep. Practicing better sleep hygiene revolves around building daily habits that provide some structure to your routine. Some helpful tips include:

- Keep a consistent bedtime and wake up at the same time each day, even on holidays and weekends.

- Keep exposure to bright lights to a minimum in the evenings, and turn off your screens (TV, phone, etc.) thirty minutes before going to bed.

- If you're not asleep after twenty minutes, get out of bed for a moment to "reset."

- Keep bedtime snacks light, and don't eat a meal late in the evening.

- Your bed should be used only for sleep and sex.

- Avoid caffeine in the afternoons or evenings.

- Avoid alcohol and limit fluids before bed, and use the bathroom before bedtime.

If you're still struggling, some therapists have specific training with insomnia and may be able to help you get to the core of the problem. Natural sleep aids are also available, like melatonin, lavender oil, or valerian root.

Melatonin is a hormone produced by the body to promote sleep. It has been studied the most frequently and has been shown to promote a natural circadian rhythm by introducing more of the hormone your body is already producing each night. A review of multiple studies published in the Journal of Neurology finds melatonin to be beneficial for improving sleep quality in many individuals experiencing insomnia. If you try melatonin, pay attention to how you feel in the morning. If you got the amount of sleep you wanted but you still feel groggy, some adjustments may be needed!

Food Follies and Hormonal Hurdles

It's no secret that diet affects the way we feel, as well as our overall well-being. We often feel these effects more directly, such as a sudden boost of energy or the tightening in our waistline that many of us experience during a holiday season filled with family and feasts. Some changes are less direct, however, and can influence our relationship with food in ways we may not realize.

Eating a diet with a lot of processed foods high in added sugars and saturated fats can raise the risk of a variety of health disorders. A primary concern of many researchers over time has been a link between trans fats and cardiovascular disease. This has led to a widespread response of regulations on food manufacturers, with the Harvard School of Public Health reporting many initiatives have made a significant impact on trans fats being used in the American food supply. While potentially a step in the right direction, what is becoming increasingly apparent are the benefits of greatly limiting or moving away from processed foods altogether.

The pitfalls of processed foods are numerous. They generally provide a lot of calories while giving you relatively few nutrients (low-calorie, nutrient-dense foods are your friend when you're trying to lose weight). Both saturated fats and sugar also contribute to the formation of fat tissue. Food with added sugars is often found with limited ingredients that help regulate potential spikes from the sugar. These ingredients are those that include nutrients such as fiber.

Processed foods can affect hormones as well; the American Journal of Clinical Nutrition highlights a clear association between dietary sugar and hormonal imbalances.

Over the years, researchers have come to understand that fat is more than simply a vessel for energy storage. It's an organ that both sends and receives signals to and from the rest of the body. These signals are—you guessed it—hormones. Leptin provides a good example of the kind of hormonal imbalance that can develop in a sneakier fashion.

Leptin is a hormone that is used by our bodies as a signal that we are full and no longer need to eat. It's produced by fat cells. The more fat cells you have, the more leptin will be circulating. So in theory, you should be less hungry, right? But in reality, your body responds to these consistently elevated levels of leptin by developing a resistance that is somewhat similar to insulin resistance. When leptin is "ignored," you may ultimately become hungrier.

The nutrients we eat are also crucial for supplying the building blocks our bodies need to keep functioning. When testosterone is produced, its building blocks are supported by your diet. In a review of multiple studies published in the Journal of Steroid Biochemistry and Molecular Biology, low-fat diets were associated with lower levels of testosterone. Which means that we can't simply stop eating dietary fats.

So, how do we achieve balance?

The answer lies in the different types of fat, because not all fats are created equal. Eating lean meats can limit saturated fats, and healthy unsaturated fats can be provided by eating foods like avocados or fish. Shifting from processed foods to whole foods removes harmful additives and retains or improves nutritional content. You're getting more beneficial nutrients from whole grains, like whole wheat and brown rice, than you would be with white bread or white rice.

Not all sugars are created equal, either. Much of what is added in sugary drinks, like sodas, and many processed baked goods has a much higher fructose content than what occurs in natural foods. This fructose content is what has primarily been associated with health concerns. There are sugars in fruits, but this doesn't mean you should avoid fresh fruit because these are natural sugars.

Some specific foods can also be added to promote hormone balance, such as flaxseed, blueberries, cherries, grapefruit, apples, and broccoli. Many of these contain flavonoids that can support testosterone production.

Staying hydrated is also crucial for maintaining healthy bodily function, including steroid production. The recommended amount of water for most men is about 3.7 liters per day—that's about 125 ounces. Keep in mind you will be getting some water from other beverages and some of the foods you eat (watermelon is aptly named as it is primarily water). Drink when you feel thirsty, and make sure your urine is clear or light yellow rather than dark yellow.

Achieving hormonal balance through diet involves limiting processed foods, choosing healthy fats like those found in avocados and fish, and incorporating nutrient-dense whole foods like fruits, vegetables, and whole grains. Staying hydrated is also key for supporting overall bodily functions, including hormone production. By making mindful food choices and maintaining a balanced diet, you can promote hormonal harmony and support your overall well-being.

The Overworked, the Overwhelmed, and the Hormonally Imbalanced

If you work an eight-hour shift and you're getting enough sleep, about half of your waking hours will be spent working on any given workday. Factor in commutes, overtime, and those times you answer the phone or an email outside of regular work hours, and the time devoted to work may be even more significant. There is little wonder that the concept of work-life balance has become so commonly discussed. For many, work *is* life.

You may love what you do, but the potential for stressors to add up is still there. No job is "perfect." Burnout, overworking, and overexertion, whether physical or mental, can creep in if we don't look honestly at our relationship with work. This is particularly true in a culture that values hard work. There is a fear that taking a breather may be seen as a sign of weakness rather than a sign of emotional intelligence. The truth is the work you do and the value you provide to your community are likely improved when you feel balanced.

Beyond not doing your performance any favors, overworking isn't doing your health any favors either. When you're stressed, you're less likely to get quality sleep and more likely to eat junk food. You may even be more likely to choose harmful coping mechanisms like drinking too much alcohol. All of these things can disrupt hormonal balance. In a study published in the Journal of Occupational and Environmental Medicine, working long hours was associated with decreased testosterone levels (Hu 2016). There have also been several studies that highlighted the pitfalls of sleep disturbances, including research that shows a strong link between shift work during non-traditional hours and lower testosterone.

Finding ways to promote better balance at work may feel like a daunting task, but there are plenty of steps you can take. For starters, make sure you are actually taking a break. We've all worked straight through a lunch break and taken quick bites of a sandwich between tasks. Take the time to sit down, away from your workstation, and actually take a break.

Learn breathing and relaxation techniques. These can be done anywhere, anytime, and many of them only take a few moments. Think of it as a "micro-break," or taking a few moments to gather yourself before diving back in. Examples include the following:

- Deep belly breathing: Breathe in slowly through your nose, allowing your belly to expand. Hold briefly, then exhale slowly through pursed lips.

- 4-7-8 breathing: Inhale for 4 counts, hold for 7 counts, exhale for 8 counts.

- Box breathing: Inhale for 4 counts, hold for 4 counts, exhale for 4 counts, hold for 4 counts. Repeat.

- Alternate nostril breathing: Use your thumb and ring finger to alternately close one nostril while inhaling through the other.

Use your vacation days. A study published in the Journal of Occupational Health describes improvements in health and well-being, including stress reduction, that result from breaks away from work, but this same study also states these improvements can be somewhat transient (Hu 2016). This highlights the importance of taking time off regularly and allowing yourself to reset.

Even if you don't plan on traveling, take a day or two to leisurely get up in the morning, go for a walk, read a book, meet a friend or family member for lunch, or spend some time on a hobby. Your time is valuable. Spend it doing something that leaves you feeling refreshed rather than drained.

The Hormonal Harmony Hijacker

Relationships with alcohol are fairly complex and varied, but like with many things, it's important to be honest with ourselves about its impact on our lives. Some studies show that certain drinks can be helpful if drinking is kept light or done in moderation. Drinks that provide polyphenols, like red wine, have been linked with a lower risk of cardiovascular disease and stroke. Of course, there are also a myriad of studies and statistics related to the downsides. There are an estimated 14 million Americans with confirmed alcoholism or habits that constitute alcohol abuse. Heavy drinkers have an increased risk of cardiovascular disease and stroke, liver disease, and many types of cancer.

Many of us are aware of these concerns and ultimately try to make healthy choices. What we don't see mentioned as frequently are the effects alcohol can have on the endocrine system—the network of hormonal messengers that govern healthy bodily functions.

Alcohol abuse has a two-fold impact on hormones. Existing hormones are not processed as efficiently by the liver, and signaling pathways leading to the production of hormones are also negatively impacted. An important example of this is the hypothalamic-pituitary-gonadal axis, which is ultimately responsible for regulating the levels of sex hormones, like testosterone, and maintaining reproductive health. Partially through a reduction of testosterone, we see memory and mood problems, decreased bone density, less muscle mass, and more fat mass developing in the longer term.

Maintaining a healthy diet is also made more difficult, depending on your drink of choice. Beer is a significant source of calories, and these can add up quickly if you're not careful. Regardless of the source of alcohol, lowered inhibitions and a tendency to reach for junk food while drinking can sabotage an otherwise healthy diet.

Limiting alcohol can be beneficial, and there are many ways to do this. Replace alcohol with another beverage, schedule drink-free days each week, or set specific goals and track your drinks on a calendar. The American Heart Association recommends no more than one or two drinks per day for men. Take an honest look at how much you drink. You want your food and beverage choices to keep you moving, not hold you back. By making conscious choices about alcohol, you can support your body's hormonal processes and promote optimal health.

Chapter Four

Food, the Fuel of Manhood

"*Let food be thy medicine and medicine be thy food.*"
- Hippocrates

Understanding the Diet-Hormone Link

We have a tendency at times to think of food as little more than a source of energy. When we're hungry, we're tired, it's harder to focus, and we may even be a bit irritable. Having a snack or a meal can get you back on your feet again. The nutrients our food choices provide (or fail to provide) may fade into an afterthought as we reach for something convenient to keep moving throughout the day.

We often attach an expectation to the medicine we've just taken for a particular ailment, in that we use it for a purpose and expect it to act in our bodies in a way that aligns with our intent. Nutrients can be thought of in a similar way. Our foods can be chosen with an intent that extends beyond an energy source for the next few hours.

Every time we eat, we have an opportunity to provide our bodies with the nutrients that become the building blocks for healthy bones and muscles. These foods can protect our hearts rather than raise the risk for cardiovascular disease. They can lay the foundation for a more efficient metabolism and influence hormone production.

The connection between food choices and blood sugar balance is an example we're all likely aware of. Eating more processed foods high in fats and sugars leaves insulin less able to manage the load. Insulin resistance develops, and blood sugars are less able to be processed effectively. Unwanted weight then has a tendency to add up. Blood sugar levels continue to build in the bloodstream, potentially leading to type 2 diabetes. Dietary choices heavily influence the potential for insulin imbalances.

Diet, stress, and hormones are also linked in a delicate dance that has the potential to stray off-kilter. There's a give-and-take here, and each of these factors has the capacity to influence the others.

Unchecked stress can lead to poor food choices. We may seek comfort or a quick meal because time needs to be devoted to more pressing matters. The meals we choose have the potential to provide nutrients that have a lasting positive impact on neurotransmitters like serotonin or provide antioxidants that improve our ability to respond to stress. Unfortunately, most convenient foods are often the least likely to provide these lasting benefits. Our recognition of this in and of itself can lead to more stress, if we don't feel empowered to make other choices. Chronic stress can lead to excessive cortisol production, which in turn affects other hormones. Some of these hormones directly affect our desire to eat.

There's a potential cycle occurring here where these factors feed into one another, and it's easy to see how the effects can build. Fortunately, there are plenty of ways to promote balance. A great place to start can be as simple as taking stock of what's in your refrigerator.

Foods That Support Hormonal Health

If you've spent much time researching dietary advice, you've likely come across some general themes. These have a tendency to be condensed into broad statements like "sugar is bad" and "fats should be limited." There is some truth to these, but generally speaking, it's those sugars and fats that are added during processing that are largely to blame for many concerns. The naturally occurring sugars in fruits shouldn't be a cause for avoiding them, although you may need to track these sugars if you are managing diabetes. Many raw fruits also offer beneficial vitamins, minerals, and phytonutrients, and their sugar content is unlikely to cause concern if they're eaten in moderation along with a balanced diet. Dietary fat provides crucial building blocks for healthy hormone production.

Supermarkets vary in their design approaches, but the general advice is to stick to the outer perimeter and limit your purchases from the inner aisles. This means focusing on fresh produce and fresh cuts from the meat counter while limiting processed foods or items with a lot of additives.

So stock up on fruits and vegetables. Raw fruits are a great way to replace otherwise unhealthy snacks and are loaded with beneficial nutrients. Many vegetables are nutrient-dense, relatively low-calorie, and can provide a number of health benefits. For instance, cruciferous vegetables like broccoli and Brussels sprouts have elevated levels of the plant steroid indole-3-carbinol. Studies have shown this has been beneficial for regulating levels of estrogen and protecting against certain types of cancer.

In a systematic review of multiple studies, men who eat low-fat diets were found to have lower levels of testosterone on average. As a reminder, simply restricting your fat intake may lead to imbalance, so the best way to address this is to take charge of the kinds of fats your diet provides. The meats you choose are a great opportunity to do this. Lean meats limit saturated fat, and foods like salmon can be great sources of healthy fats like omega-3 fatty acids. These fats help with hormone production and can help protect against cardiovascular disease.

Sources of carbohydrates, like grains, are generally better for you the less processed they are. For instance, white rice is produced by removing the outer bran layer. This results in a loss of beneficial nutrients, fiber, and other bioactive compounds. Brown rice retains these nutrients. Whole grain products, like whole wheat bread, follow the same concept.

A primary benefit of whole grains is the dietary fiber. We have a tendency to think of digestive health first when considering fiber, but the benefits extend beyond keeping things moving in the digestive tract. Dietary fiber has been associated with improvements in metabolism. These improvements are linked to blood sugar control, insulin balance, and weight management.

Fiber also supports a healthy balance of gut microbiota, which are the beneficial bacteria living in your gut. Research is developing in several areas within gut health, ranging from potential benefits for local inflammation and immune response to the concept of a gut-brain axis. Healthy gut bacteria may promote better responses to stress, which means there may be improvements in mood for individuals managing anxiety or depression. Gut bacteria have the potential to influence overall health in ways we are just beginning to understand. Fiber provides fuel for these beneficial bacteria to thrive.

So, how can we put all of this together? Ultimately, individual dietary needs may differ depending on medical status, and major changes are always best discussed with your doctor. The ideal place to start is by taking the time to give your food the thought it deserves. What nutrients are your meals providing? Are there opportunities to improve individual components by limiting saturated fats with leaner cuts or by introducing additional nutrients with whole grains? At times, the simplest way to begin improving your diet is to identify those foods that may be the most harmful and find ways to limit or remove them.

Foods to Avoid for Optimal Hormone Health

When pressed with the question, "What did you eat today?" many of us have a tendency to forget one of the more insidious sources of sugar and empty calories: beverages. In the United States, it's estimated that over half of the population drinks at least one soft drink (i.e., soda, pop, coke, etc.) every day. A portion of these individuals drink three or four (or more) soft drinks daily.

So, let's do some quick math. A typical soda contains about 150 calories. One soda per day works out to about 1,050 calories per week, provided with little or no nutritional value. Three sodas per day would increase that weekly total to around 3,150 calories. Losing weight is dependent on burning more calories than you consume. The caloric deficit needed to lose one pound of body weight varies between individuals, but a rough estimate of about 3,500 calories per pound can be used. This means switching from soda to water could promote weight loss of nearly a pound per week for those who drink several sodas daily.

Of course, due to the large amounts of readily available sugar in these drinks, there are significant spikes and crashes in blood sugar levels. These crashes can leave you tired and irritable, potentially craving more. This also places a strain on insulin and our body's metabolism, which can lead to imbalances over time. Fruit juices often have added sugars and tend to have the same effect.

Unfortunately, diet sodas don't necessarily solve this problem either. In a study published in Trends in Endocrinology and Metabolism, the artificial sweeteners used in diet sodas were found to impact metabolism in ways that actually promote weight gain (Jones 2006). The risks of developing type 2 diabetes and heart disease remain elevated with artificial sweetener use.

Many foods share this problem and often take things a step beyond added sugar by adding saturated fats and high salt levels. Some of these flavors are delicious, and craving them becomes almost second nature over time. These saturated fats can contribute to insulin and energy imbalances as well. Both the fats and the high salt levels contribute to the risk of cardiovascular disease by increasing inflammation, plaque buildup in arteries, and raising blood pressure.

Heavily processed foods check all these boxes, but there are also some sources of additives that may not be as readily apparent. For instance, certain lunch meats and sausages can be particularly high in salt and fat content. Breakfast cereals have the potential to add a lot of sugar, depending on your choice, despite being marketed as a healthy breakfast alternative. Prepackaged dried fruits are often loaded with added salt and sugar. Foods labeled "fat-free" are often loaded with alternative additives to avoid becoming bland. It can be helpful to take a moment to consider how the foods you buy at the grocery store are prepared before they make their way into your cart.

Preparing more meals at home also gives you control over the ingredients. Eating out can be a great way to get out and connect with people, but there are some pitfalls. Meals at many sit-down restaurants are delicious in part due to a significant amount of butter. This versatile ingredient is a staple in professional kitchens, enhancing flavors and textures in ways that home cooks often underestimate. Chefs use butter liberally to create rich sauces, achieve perfectly browned meats, and add a silky finish to vegetables. In pasta dishes, a pat of butter can transform a simple sauce into a luxurious coating, while in baking, it contributes to the flakiness of pastries and the tenderness of cakes. Even in savory dishes where butter isn't the star, it's often used to sauté aromatics, adding depth to the foundation of the meal. This generous use of butter in restaurant cooking is one of the reasons why dishes often taste more indulgent and satisfying than their home-cooked counterparts. However, it's also why restaurant meals tend to be higher in calories and saturated fats, making them less suitable for everyday consumption for those mindful of their dietary intake.

While butter can make food taste great, consuming large amounts regularly can have negative health implications. Butter is high in saturated fat, which has been linked to an increase in LDL cholesterol levels (often called "bad cholesterol") when consumed in excess. Elevated LDL cholesterol is a risk factor for heart disease and stroke. Additionally, the high calorie content of butter can contribute to weight gain if not balanced with overall calorie needs and physical activity. Diets high in saturated fats have also been associated with increased inflammation in the body, which is linked to various chronic diseases. The high sodium content often found in restaurant meals, partially due to the salted butter used in cooking, can also contribute to high blood pressure in some individuals. It's worth noting that while moderate butter consumption can be part of a balanced diet, the amounts used in restaurant cooking often exceed recommended daily intakes. This is why nutrition experts often advise limiting restaurant meals and preparing more foods at home, where you can control the amount of butter and other high-fat ingredients used in cooking.

Culturally, we expect large portion sizes in exchange for our money. Take-out and drive-thru meals are convenient, but eating these meals consistently can begin to create nutrient imbalances. A study published in the Journal of the Academy of Nutrition and Dietetics found that fewer than one in five meals served at popular restaurants met nutritional criteria set forth by the American Heart Association (Alexander 2020). This is to say, ultimately, many of these meals may increase the risk of cardiovascular disease.

Alcohol is also important to consider. Studies link excessive drinking with lower levels of testosterone and sperm counts (along with a number of other health concerns). Take the time to inventory your alcohol intake, as sometimes these drinks can add up more quickly than we realize. Alcohol can also impact judgment and create setbacks in other areas related to nutrition, so awareness and moderation are important.

These cycles can be broken by replacing some of the repeat offenders in our diets with healthier choices. Taking a few steps in the right direction can help you build long-lasting habits over time, and these healthy habits can pay dividends for years to come.

Making Hormone-Friendly Dietary Changes

We've all come across plenty of trendy diets. We may have even tried a few at one time or another. Social media and websites dedicated to health tips are full of detox plans, tight schedules, and restrictive diets. Many of these represent a fundamental change in our habits and can be difficult (or even unhealthy) to follow consistently for a period longer than a week or two. In many cases, we lose water weight quickly, experience weight loss plateaus, life moves on, and potentially, that weight comes right back. While some plans do hold some merit, all too often, no meaningful changes occur in the long term.

So, how do you build meaningful change? What are some changes that will support your health long-term by supporting a healthy metabolism, keeping hormones balanced, and keeping body fat in check? Put simply, changing everything all at once can be an unrealistic approach. We are creatures of habit, and those habits are built over time. Incremental changes may feel small, but they can be built upon and have lasting effects if we stick with them over time.

Thinking back to those foods that are best avoided, the next step is to take some time to identify what they can be replaced with. In some instances, this becomes a question of time management. Have specific meals and snacks in mind when you shop for groceries, prepare them ahead of time, and limit your trips to vending machines, gas station snack aisles, and fast food restaurants. This can ultimately save time, money, and improve your overall health. Many pitfalls lie in convenience, and a little planning can go a long way.

Here's a list of foods that men should consider avoiding or limiting for balanced hormonal health:

1. Processed Foods:

- High in trans fats, refined sugars, and artificial additives.

- Can disrupt hormone balance and increase inflammation.

2. Excessive Alcohol:

- Can lower testosterone levels and increase estrogen.

- Impacts liver function, which is crucial for hormone metabolism.

3. Soy Products (in large quantities):

- Contains phytoestrogens that may affect testosterone levels.

- Moderation is key; small amounts are generally fine.

4. Sugar and Refined Carbohydrates:

- Can lead to insulin resistance and hormonal imbalances.

- May contribute to weight gain, which affects hormone levels.

5. Non-Organic Dairy and Meat:

- May contain added hormones that can disrupt natural hormone balance.

- Opt for organic or hormone-free options when possible.

6. High-Mercury Fish:

- Mercury can interfere with hormone production and function.

- Limit consumption of large predatory fish like shark, swordfish, and king mackerel.

7. Artificial Sweeteners:

- May disrupt gut bacteria, potentially affecting hormone regulation.

- Can lead to increased cravings and metabolic issues.

8. Excessive Caffeine:

- Can increase cortisol levels and disrupt sleep patterns.

- Moderation is key; limit to one-two cups of coffee per day.

9. Licorice Root (in large amounts):

- Can lower testosterone levels.

- Avoid regular consumption of licorice root supplements or excessive licorice candy.

10. Mint and Peppermint:

- May lower testosterone levels if consumed in large quantities.

- Moderation is key; occasional consumption is generally fine.

11. Canned Foods:

- Often lined with BPA, which can disrupt hormone function.

- Choose fresh or frozen alternatives when possible.

12. Microwaved Popcorn:

- The bag lining often contains chemicals that can disrupt hormones.

- Opt for air-popped or stovetop popcorn instead.

13. Vegetable Oils High in Omega-6:

- Excessive consumption can lead to inflammation and hormonal imbalances.

- Limit use of corn, soybean, and sunflower oils.

14. Excessively Charred Meats:

- Can contain compounds that interfere with hormone production.

- Avoid burning or charring meats when cooking.

15. Artificial Food Coloring:

- May contain endocrine disruptors.

- Choose naturally colored foods and beverages.

Moderation is key for most of these foods. A balanced diet that includes a variety of whole foods is generally the best approach for maintaining hormonal health. Realistically, there are times when life does make this difficult, with schedules and obligations building up. Looking for opportunities to swap out relatively unhealthy foods with healthier options can make a big difference over time. It's okay to start small and build on it.

Being more mindful of snacks and beverages can be a great place to start. For example, switching processed snacks to a handful of almonds is an easy way to add some nutritional value. Almonds are an excellent source of vitamin E and healthy fats that support hormone production. Fresh fruit can satisfy a sweet tooth by providing natural sugar along with many crucial vitamins and minerals. Swap caffeinated sodas and energy drinks for coffee or tea. Switch from sugary drinks to flavored sparkling water or just plain water.

Ingredients can be swapped out in meals, or alternative side dishes can be used to help provide key nutrients while limiting unhealthy fat, salt, and sugar. For instance, grains form the basis of many meals, so swapping brown rice for white rice allows you to take advantage of the full nutritional value of rice. This includes plenty of fiber, which can help regulate digestive health and blood sugar metabolism. Whole-grain breads offer a similar advantage over white bread. Oatmeal or a fruit parfait are great replacements for heavily processed breakfast cereals.

Tracking these changes over time gives you an opportunity to take stock of how the benefits they offer have affected you. Seeing changes in your weight can help you stay motivated, but there are also some potential changes that are harder to quantify. Keeping notes in a journal or using an app to track your progress over time can also help you identify broader changes in energy levels and mood. It's also always a good idea to consult with a healthcare professional or a registered dietitian for personalized dietary advice.

As you make modifications to the way your pantry is stocked over time and develop a tendency to choose healthier options over the course of the day, habits develop. Eating healthier can become second nature, rather than the uphill battle we may feel we face initially.

Here are fifteen hormone-friendly recipes for men that are easy to make with common ingredients:

1. Grilled Salmon with Lemon and Dill:

- Rich in omega-3 fatty acids and vitamin D.

- Ingredients: salmon filet, lemon, dill, olive oil, salt, pepper.

2. Spinach and Mushroom Frittata:

- High in protein and zinc.

- Ingredients: eggs, spinach, mushrooms, onion, cheese, olive oil.

3. Avocado and Tuna Salad:

- Good source of healthy fats and protein.

- Ingredients: canned tuna, avocado, red onion, lemon juice, olive oil.

4. Grilled Chicken with Roasted Vegetables:

- Lean protein and nutrient-rich veggies.

- Ingredients: chicken breast, bell peppers, zucchini, onion, olive oil, herbs.

5. Overnight Oats with Berries and Nuts:

- High in fiber and healthy fats.

- Ingredients: oats, milk (or plant-based alternative), berries, nuts, honey.

6. Lentil and Vegetable Soup:

- Rich in fiber and plant-based protein.

- Ingredients: lentils, carrots, celery, onion, garlic, vegetable broth, spices.

7. Stir-Fried Tofu with Broccoli:

- Good source of plant-based protein and cruciferous vegetables.

- Ingredients: firm tofu, broccoli, garlic, ginger, soy sauce, sesame oil.

8. Greek Yogurt Parfait:

- High in protein and probiotics.

- Ingredients: greek yogurt, granola, mixed berries, honey.

9. Baked Sweet Potato with Black Beans:

- Rich in complex carbs and plant-based protein.

- Ingredients: sweet potato, black beans, salsa, avocado, cilantro.

10. Grilled Grass-Fed Beef Skewers:

- Excellent source of protein and zinc.

- Ingredients: beef cubes, bell peppers, onion, olive oil, herbs.

11. Quinoa and Vegetable Stir-Fry:

- Complete protein source with added vegetables.

- Ingredients: quinoa, mixed vegetables, garlic, ginger, soy sauce.

12. Sardine and Avocado Toast:

- Rich in omega-3 fatty acids and healthy fats.

- Ingredients: whole grain bread, canned sardines, avocado, lemon juice.

13. Turkey and Vegetable Chili:

- Lean protein with fiber-rich beans.

- Ingredients: ground turkey, kidney beans, tomatoes, onion, bell peppers, chili spices.

14. Baked Cod with Tomatoes and Olives:

- Lean protein with Mediterranean flavors.

- Ingredients: cod filet, cherry tomatoes, olives, garlic, olive oil, herbs.

15. Pumpkin Seed and Berry Smoothie:

- Rich in zinc and antioxidants.

- Ingredients: pumpkin seeds, mixed berries, spinach, Greek yogurt, almond milk.

These recipes are designed to support hormonal health with ingredients rich in essential nutrients like zinc, omega-3 fatty acids, fiber, and lean proteins. They're also relatively simple to prepare, making it easier to maintain a hormone-friendly diet. Adjust portions and ingredients based on individual dietary needs and preferences.

As we've explored the nutritional component of hormone health, we've uncovered a powerful truth: the foods we choose to eat—and those we decide to avoid—play a crucial role in maintaining hormonal balance. By embracing a diet rich in whole foods, lean proteins, healthy fats, and plenty of fruits and vegetables, while limiting processed foods, excessive sugar, and hormone-disrupting substances, you can take significant strides toward optimal hormonal health. Remember, small, consistent changes in your diet can lead to substantial improvements in your overall well-being and hormonal balance over time.

However, nutrition is just one piece of the puzzle when it comes to hormonal health. Another critical, yet often overlooked, factor is hydration. As we transition to our next section on the importance of hydration in men's hormonal health, we'll discover how proper fluid intake goes far beyond simply quenching thirst. Adequate hydration is fundamental to numerous bodily functions, including hormone production, transportation, and metabolism. It also plays a vital role in maintaining healthy body composition, which directly impacts hormone levels. So, let's dive into the refreshing world of hydration and uncover how this simple, everyday practice can have profound effects on your hormonal health and overall vitality.

Staying Hydrated: an Essential Aspect of Hormonal Health

We're likely all familiar with dehydration as a potential source of more immediate concern. Becoming light-headed while working outside, sweating on a particularly hot day, or watching for signs of dehydration in our children while they manage diarrhea. The context is often fluid loss and the need to replace it.

Under more normal circumstances, we see the recommendations for the amount of water we should be drinking every day, but in the absence of an emergency, some of the finer points may get lost in the background. Estimates vary widely, but it has been suggested as many as three out of four adults in the United States are chronically dehydrated. The body responds to fluid and electrolyte imbalances through a variety of systems, and ultimately, a lack of hydration places stress on a number of different functions.

There is a direct link between lack of hydration and blood pressure control, as well as broader concerns related to higher risks of developing cardiovascular disease. The body has to work actively to maintain normal blood pressure and levels of electrolytes. Much of this activity is regulated by the sympathetic nervous system, stress hormones like cortisol, and hormones that manage electrolytes like aldosterone. The need for these hormones to work overtime can create imbalances.

When dehydration becomes an emergency, there is ultimately a relative failure of the body to compensate. Someone could lose consciousness, for instance. The heart is pounding, trying to compensate for lower blood volumes and keep the body supplied with oxygen. Our bodies do a good job of compensating before an emergency situation arises, but a constant need to compensate can take its toll over time. Because of this, chronic dehydration becomes a long-term health concern.

Broader recommendations trend toward about eight 8-ounce glasses of water each day. That is 1.89 liters or about 64 ounces. Other recommendations call for a total of 3.7 liters each day from all sources (including food, which is estimated to provide about 20 percent of our daily water).

Recommendations for staying hydrated become somewhat muddy because of a variety of factors. We have variable levels of physical activity and ways of losing water. Kidney function can vary. Some individuals take diuretics to treat high blood pressure, causing them to lose more water in urine. Our body size and composition—the amount of fat and muscle we have—varies between individuals. The foods we eat contain different amounts of water (the weight of fresh fruits and vegetables is often primarily water). In reality, there is no one-size-fits-all magic amount of water each of us should be drinking each day.

In practical terms, being mindful of fluid intake may be more beneficial than tracking your water down to the ounce. Drink a glass of water with each meal and another between meals. Drink water before, during, and after exercise or while working outside and sweating because you're likely to lose more fluids during these times. Drink water when you feel thirsty, and monitor your urine. Colorless or light yellow is what you want to see; if it's dark yellow, drink some water.

The Role of Micronutrients in Hormonal Health

When approaching a diet, we tend to spend the majority of our time thinking about macronutrients. Our diets are composed of several macronutrients, and these are broadly defined as proteins, fats, and carbohydrates. Of course, there are different types of carbohydrates—simple and complex, for instance—and different types of fats—saturated and unsaturated—with certain foods providing healthier sources of these types than others. Macronutrients make up the primary sources of calories because they can be directly broken down to provide energy.

However, our nutritional needs extend into broader sources of energy, and micronutrients fill these roles. They are "micro" in that they are provided in fairly small amounts, but their absence can have far-reaching effects on our health. These are the vitamins and minerals our bodies need to perform many basic functions, including hormone production.

Vitamin D is involved in testosterone production, and lower levels of vitamin D are linked with low levels of testosterone. Low levels of vitamin D are also associated with broader concerns like cardiovascular disease and depression. Zinc is a crucial component of many enzymes that contribute to a range of processes in the body. Its impact ranges from immune response to hormone production.

Fortunately, many of the foods that provide healthier sources of macronutrients are also rich in micronutrients. Foods like salmon provide healthy fats and are a good source of vitamin D. Zinc can be found in seafood, legumes (i.e., beans), and seeds, among other sources.

Quality foods provide quality nutrients. A balanced diet with sources of lean protein, healthy fats, and complex carbohydrates paired with fiber will generally provide all the micronutrients you need. Fresh, unprocessed foods are also often more nutrient-dense, providing more beneficial vitamins and minerals without loading up on calories.

Nutrient deficiencies can occur for a variety of reasons, and regularly checking in with your doctor can help you identify these. Your doctor can help you identify potential causes and work with you to develop a personalized plan. For those times when supplements are recommended, they can help fill the gaps and get you back on track.

Navigating the Maze of Diet Trends

During a meet-up with a friend, the topic of conversation landed on intermittent fasting—it turned out they had lost twenty pounds and counting! A family member recently tried the keto diet and raved about how great they feel. If you express an interest in healthy eating and scroll through social media, there are products, plans, and promises as far as the eye can see.

Social media, healthcare blogs, articles, friends, and family—we tend to hear a lot of information about potential diet plans from a lot of different sources. The thing is, we *want* these approaches to work for others, in part because it makes us feel like we can do it, too. These before and after images are exciting. They are motivating.

The truth is many trendy diets can offer some very legitimate merits, but it's important to recognize the potential differences in how individuals respond to these approaches. What works well for some may be dangerous for others.

The keto diet is a good example of this. Essentially, it takes a high-protein, low-carbohydrate diet to a more restrictive extreme, leading to the body transitioning away from glucose as a primary energy source in favor of ketones. This can be very dangerous for individuals with an existing metabolic imbalance like diabetes. Ketoacidosis is a life-threatening condition requiring emergency care, and purposefully increasing ketones can make this more likely. For many, a delicate balance needs to be maintained, and achieving it is much more likely with the help of a doctor, dietitian, or both.

Intermittent fasting is meant to induce a period of fat-burning on a daily basis. It can also increase levels of cortisol and ultimately impact other hormones, like testosterone, negatively if approached too aggressively.

As certain food groups are restricted, certain nutrients become more scarce. This opens up the potential for deficiencies. Restrictive diets are also notoriously difficult to maintain long-term, and "yo-yo dieting" may actually be more harmful than altering your diet in the first place.

Your current health status should always be taken into consideration. Before starting any new diet, particularly one that places heavy restrictions, it's always best to talk with a healthcare provider. Each of us has individual needs, and a healthcare team, including a functional medicine practitioner or registered dietitian, can help you identify a more detailed, personalized plan based on your health and goals moving forward.

Chapter Five

Harnessing Nature's Pharmacy for Hormone Balance

Understanding the Role of Natural and Herbal Products in Hormone Balance

The over-the-counter supplement market is booming, fueled by a desire to seek natural approaches to health that either augment or replace treatment options. Many men utilize a wide range of natural products to support various areas of wellness. It's important to take some time to familiarize yourself with what's out there. What do some of these ingredients do, what is their place in an overall approach to wellness, and what risks are important to be aware of?

The role of many nutritional supplements can be broadly defined as prevention. This can mean preventing nutritional gaps related to key nutrients or attempting to lower the risk for diseases like cancer or heart disease. Many supplements also provide ingredients that play a role in supporting healthy hormone production.

In some instances, benefits have the potential to go beyond addressing or avoiding nutritional deficits. For example, ashwagandha, an herb used in Ayurvedic medicine (a traditional approach to medicine developed over 3,000 years ago in India), has been associated with reduced levels of cortisol. This has the potential to translate to improved stress management and may help prevent the disruption of other hormones caused by chronic elevations of cortisol.

As time goes on and traditional approaches to medicine become studied more extensively with modern methods, variability in responses between individuals becomes more apparent. For instance, some men may find stress-related symptoms improve while using St. John's Wort, while others may be more likely to experience bothersome side effects like sensitivity to light. It's also important to consider a wide range of potential interactions with medications associated with St. John's Wort, most notably prescriptions commonly prescribed for anxiety and depression. If you are already under existing medical care, it's crucial to discuss each aspect of your therapy to ensure safety.

Prevention is a main focus of a more natural approach. If there is an existing imbalance, it's always best addressed with individualized help from a healthcare professional. Consulting with a provider before starting a new supplement gives you an opportunity to review how it may interact with your current health or treatments.

It's important to remember that natural products can provide support, but they are not able to replace a healthy balanced diet, adequate sleep, and regular exercise. These are the cornerstones of hormonal health and represent a necessity within any successful holistic approach. Taking these areas for granted sabotages your efforts elsewhere, leaving you with an uphill battle. Supplements are not a magic solution but rather a complementary tool to support overall wellness when used responsibly and in conjunction with a healthy lifestyle.

Digging Deeper: a Spotlight on Key Natural Products for Hormonal Health

Navigating the over-the-counter supplement market can become confusing rather quickly. There are a potentially overwhelming number of ingredients combined in countless formulations, and new products become available frequently. Marketing techniques often employ unapologetic hype but can also provide references to clinical studies meant to support health claims.

These studies add some clout, and when they're linked directly, they can add helpful transparency. However, it's also important to consider the quality of the studies used to back these statements. For instance, studies conducted in humans provide better insight compared with animal models. Studies conducted using cell lines or test tubes identifying a proposed mechanism of benefit are more helpful for guiding future studies than they are for directly predicting how your body will respond. As consumers of these products, we want results. We want to know how much to take, how much of a difference it will make, and whether there are potential side effects to be aware of.

Prospective, blinded, randomized, placebo-controlled trials better establish cause and effect compared with retrospective chart reviews or broad surveys requiring participants to recall past events. Meta-analyses that combine the results of multiple trials can provide even more insight, in part due to their larger aggregate sample size. Larger studies carry more weight than small studies.

If you have an interest in following up on some of the claims you see listed on supplement websites or product packaging, these basic tenets can give you a better grasp of the quality of evidence. Ultimately, additional research is needed for many natural products to give a definitive picture of the overall potential benefits. However, among the myriad products marketed for men's health, several ingredients do stand out as potentially more beneficial.

Ashwagandha is worth mentioning again because it's a good example of a natural product with what could be considered above-average clinical clout. It's considered an adaptogen, which means it can help the body adapt or respond to stress. In a meta-analysis of controlled trials, ashwagandha was found to significantly reduce symptoms of anxiety and stress levels compared with a placebo, which lends some direct evidence of repeatable results. Stress management is important because unchecked stress can lead to hormonal imbalance.

Ashwagandha is usually available in capsule form, and the recommended dose can vary depending on the individual. An example of a successful dose for improved stress management in studies was 300 mg dosed twice daily for a period of 60 days.

Another example of a natural supplement with some promising study results is Tongkat Ali (sometimes referred to solely as *Eurycoma longifolia* in research). This is an herbal supplement with roots in Malaysia and has been used for hundreds of years. A meta-analysis of clinical trials has shown a positive impact on testosterone production in men. It has also been studied more specifically for erectile dysfunction and appears to offer improvements in erection quality.

Tongkat Ali is available in several forms, including powders, teas, and capsules. It's important to consult a healthcare provider to ensure safe, appropriate dosing. In one study involving men with androgen deficiencies associated with aging, a 200 mg dose was associated with improved erectile function.

Maca, a plant native to Peru, has long been associated with boosting energy, stamina, and libido. In a systematic review of its effects, maca was associated with improvements in erectile function and improvements in both male and female sexual desire.

Maca is often available in a powder form that can be added to smoothies or cereals and can also be taken as a capsule. It's important to note that the doses used in studies have varied, and further studies would be helpful in identifying an optimal dose. A study evaluating both a 1.5-gram and 3.0-gram dose found no additional benefit associated with the higher dose (Shin 2010).

So we can see that these alternatives are an appealing option for men who are seeking natural approaches to support their hormonal health—both those looking for gentler options and those who want complementary approaches to traditional medical treatments. However, it's important to approach these natural solutions with both enthusiasm and caution.

The following list presents some of the most commonly used natural remedies for men's hormonal health. Each item has been associated with potential benefits for various aspects of male hormone function, from supporting testosterone production to improving libido and overall well-being. These remedies draw from diverse traditions, including ancient herbal practices, modern nutritional science, and emerging research in men's health.

While many of these natural options show promise, it's crucial to remember that "natural" doesn't always mean "safe" or "effective" for everyone. Remember, the impact of these remedies can vary greatly between individuals, and some may interact with existing medications or health conditions. Additionally, the regulatory oversight for supplements is often less stringent than for pharmaceuticals, making quality and dosage consistency potential concerns. Before incorporating any of these remedies into your health regimen, it's essential to consult with a healthcare professional. They can provide guidance on potential benefits, risks, and appropriate usage based on your individual health profile. With that in mind, let's explore some of the most popular natural options for supporting men's hormonal health:

1. Ashwagandha:
    - Purpose: stress reduction; may increase testosterone levels.
    - Use: adaptogen that helps balance cortisol levels.

2. Zinc:
    - Purpose: supports testosterone production and sperm health.
    - Use: essential mineral for male reproductive function.

3. Vitamin D:
    - Purpose: may boost testosterone levels; supports overall hormone function.
    - Use: supplement, especially in regions with limited sunlight.

4. Fenugreek:
    - Purpose: may increase testosterone levels and libido.
    - Use: herb taken in supplement form.

5. D-Aspartic Acid:
   - Purpose: can boost testosterone production.
   - Use: amino acid supplement.

6. Maca Root:
   - Purpose: may improve libido and fertility.
   - Use: adaptogenic herb, often taken as a powder.

7. Magnesium:
   - Purpose: supports testosterone production and overall hormone balance.
   - Use: essential mineral; can be taken as a supplement.

8. Ginger:
   - Purpose: may increase testosterone levels and sperm quality.
   - Use: can be consumed as food, tea, or supplement.

9. Tribulus Terrestris:
   - Purpose: may improve libido and erectile function.
   - Use: herbal supplement.

10. Saw Palmetto:
    - Purpose: supports prostate health; may help with testosterone balance.
    - Use: herbal supplement.

11. DHEA:
    - Purpose: precursor to testosterone; may improve hormone

levels in older men.

- Use: supplement, but should be used under medical supervision.

12. Boron:
    - Purpose: may help increase free testosterone levels.
    - Use: trace mineral; can be taken as a supplement.

13. Omega-3 Fatty Acids:
    - Purpose: support overall hormone function and reduce inflammation.
    - Use: found in fish oil or algae-based supplements.

14. Tongkat Ali:
    - Purpose: may increase testosterone levels and improve libido.
    - Use: herbal supplement.

15. Panax Ginseng:
    - Purpose: may improve erectile function and increase testosterone.
    - Use: herbal supplement.

16. Chrysin:
    - Purpose: may help prevent the conversion of testosterone to estrogen.
    - Use: flavonoid supplement.

17. Indole-3-Carbinol:

- Purpose: supports healthy estrogen metabolism.

- Use: found in cruciferous vegetables; also available as a supplement.

18. Stinging Nettle Root:
    - Purpose: may support prostate health and free testosterone levels.

    - Use: herbal supplement.

The Flip Side: Understanding the Potential Risks of Natural Products

Ultimately, treatment decisions come down to an evaluation of the potential risks compared with the benefits. Regardless of whether you're using a prescription product or an over-the-counter natural supplement, there is a possibility that harm may be caused. Weighing the potential harm—and understanding what can make it more likely—is a crucial step along the path to better health.

For instance, products like Tongkat Ali can cause difficulty sleeping, particularly when taken at higher doses. A sleep disruption may ultimately outweigh the beneficial effects for some individuals. It's also important to consider potential interactions with existing therapy. As we already mentioned, St. John's Wort can be beneficial for some individuals managing stress and depression, but it should be used with caution by those using prescription medications. It can interact with antidepressants, heart medications, birth control, and other medications, highlighting the importance of consulting healthcare professionals before starting new supplements.

It's also important to be aware of inconsistencies in the quality of over-the-counter products. Using reputable brands is crucial because, unlike prescription medications, the FDA does not actively evaluate individual over-the-counter products available on the market. In a study published in the Journal of the American Medical Association, 776 dietary supplements were found to include unapproved ingredients that were not visible on the label (Tucker 2018). Among these supplements, a majority of them were marketed for sexual enhancement, weight loss, or muscle building—common goals among men concerned with hormonal balance. These ingredients have the potential to cause harm, particularly when used unknowingly. Many products have also been found to contain smaller amounts of active ingredients than indicated on the label, and some ingredients are entirely absent. While arguably less insidious, this is certainly harmful to the pocketbook.

So evaluating brands and manufacturers is important, but what are some of the best ways to do this? Many brands tout good manufacturing practices, or GMP-certified facilities, which can be a positive sign. However, it's important to clarify what this means, particularly when some manufacturers use language implying "FDA approval." Good manufacturing practices are guidelines established by the FDA to help ensure product integrity. The FDA does not give certifications; they are given by third-party companies that help manufacturers prepare for potential inspections. In this sense, the manufacturer establishes a commitment to "FDA-approved manufacturing practices," which is often used as a marketing component. As far as the FDA is directly concerned, intervention is unlikely unless a violation has occurred. Checking for a history of any FDA warning letters can help you determine whether good manufacturing practices have been a concern in the past. When companies highlight GMP certification, it's generally a positive sign but should not be mistaken for a form of FDA approval.

Arguably, submissions to independent, third-party lab testing are one of the more important signs of a quality, reliable manufacturer. These tests vary, but they can confirm that active ingredients are present in the doses advertised. Many of these tests also check for harmful contaminants that can be introduced during manufacturing.

Take some time to research the brand before you make a purchase. It's important to be aware of the potential for substantial differences in quality between manufacturers. Look for reputable brands that prioritize transparency, undergo third-party testing, and have a clean track record with regulatory agencies. While supplements can be beneficial, it's crucial to approach them with caution and due diligence to ensure you're getting a safe and effective product.

Crafting a Personalized Plan: Integrating Natural Products into Your Hormonal Health Routine

The process of integrating new natural products into your routine can be broken up into three basic steps:

- assess your individual needs,

- choose the right products, and

- actively monitor your response.

Remember, your needs are unique to you; they may differ from your friend down the street or your cousin living in Chicago. If something works well for them, that's wonderful—you still need to ensure the products you use are the right choice for *your* needs.

If you're feeling stressed, this is a primary factor to address. You may get more beneficial support from using a supplement like ashwagandha, which has shown some benefits for stress management. If you're feeling exhausted or you feel sexual dysfunction is a concern, supplements like Maca or Tongkat Ali may be more helpful for your needs. These supplements have been shown to help in different ways, so identifying your needs is crucial for maximizing the benefits you receive.

Once you've talked with a healthcare provider and determined a particular supplement is right for you, it's time to choose the product. As previously mentioned, your choice of brands matters regarding nutritional supplements. This is not like receiving generic medication from your pharmacy. Over-the-counter brands are not required to undergo rigorous testing to ensure equivalency to one another.

Brand reputation and signs of quality are important. Brands like Gaia Herbs and NOW Foods are well-known for their policies related to quality control, and they offer a wide range of products.

When you start taking a new supplement, it can be helpful to remember an old adage within medicine: "Start low and go slow." Just because these products are natural does not mean they are inert (we wouldn't be taking them if they were). These products can be potent, and allowing your body to adjust is beneficial. Increase the dose slowly over time.

It can also be helpful to take things a step further and track how you're feeling. Keep a simple daily journal to help you record changes in symptoms (including potential side effects along with those symptoms you intend to treat), energy levels, and your overall sense of well-being. This can give you a sense of how well the product may be working over time and can be particularly helpful for symptoms that may be more difficult to track, such as stress. Sometimes, symptoms are an afterthought if we're not actively managing them, so take some time to reflect.

Unlock the Power of Hormonal Health

"Understanding your body is the first step to transforming your life."
- Dr. Ashley Sullivan, PharmD

You've taken an incredible step by diving into "Understanding Hormones for Men." Now, I've got a question that might just change someone else's life:

Would you help another guy reclaim his vitality, even if you never met him or got credit for it?

If you're nodding, I've got a small but mighty request. It's for a man out there who's feeling lost, tired, and unsure about his body's changes. He's you, a few months or years ago, searching for answers and hope.

To fulfill our mission of empowering men to take control of their hormonal health, we need to reach more people like you. Since most guys judge a book by its cover (and reviews), I'm asking for a tiny favor that'll take less than a minute of your time.

Your honest review could:

• Help one more man understand his body better

• Guide someone towards regaining their energy and confidence

• Inspire a father to be more present for his family

• Change countless lives by spreading hormonal health awareness

All it takes is 60 seconds to leave a review. That's shorter than your morning shower!

Scan below to access the review page on Amazon!

P.S. If helping another guy on his hormone journey feels good, you're exactly the kind of person I love supporting. I can't wait to share more insights with you in the upcoming chapters!

P.P.S. Remember: Sharing valuable knowledge creates a ripple effect of health and happiness. Pass this book along to other men in your life who might need it.

Thank you from the bottom of my heart. Now, let's dive back into the fascinating world of hormones!

Dr. Ashley

Chapter Six

Navigating the Waves of Change: Understanding Age-Related Hormonal Shifts

"*To me, old age is always fifteen years older than I am.*"
  - Bernard Baruch, Political Consultant.

The Aging Process and Hormonal Shifts

Many changes define aging. Some of these are positive: we have an opportunity to gain from our experiences; perspective can be found more easily at times; and we can begin to enjoy the path as much as the destination. However, our bodies tend to slow down over time, contributing to that common feeling of, "If only I had known what I know now when I was younger, think of what I could have *done*!"

There's plenty more to do, of course, even if it seems our bodies move a little more slowly at times. One of the ways we discussed earlier that our bodies fundamentally change over time is a decrease in the production of sex hormones like testosterone. It's worth the reminder that starting at around age thirty to forty, testosterone levels begin to steadily decline at a rate of about 1 percent per year. This decline is an expected, natural process, but it does have the potential to become imbalanced.

As a point of interest (and perhaps concern), researchers have suggested that the levels of testosterone among American men may also be lower relative to our forefathers. There could be a number of factors at work here, but ultimately it can feel as though the cards are stacked against us in our attempts to maintain normalcy.

These changes can impact overall health and well-being significantly. Lower levels of testosterone, particularly those considered to represent an imbalance, can leave us feeling tired and irritable. They can also affect our body composition, resulting in increased body fat stores and decreased lean muscle mass. These metabolic changes can ultimately contribute to the risks of cardiovascular disease.

A certain level of testosterone decline is normal, particularly if the decreases are occurring gradually over time. A more sudden, rapid change is certainly more concerning, but all men can benefit from appropriate monitoring and routine checkups with healthcare providers over time. Awareness of the signs of potential imbalances can lead to more effective self-monitoring and conversations with your doctor. These routine checkups can help set you on a healthier course before potential imbalances blossom into bigger problems.

Recognizing the Symptoms of Age-Related Hormonal Changes

One of the trickier aspects of detecting age-related hormonal changes is the common ground shared with our perception of aging. Sometimes changes are subtle, and we can have a tendency to write them off. When it takes a bit longer to get moving before your first cup of coffee in the morning or those afternoon naps become more appealing, it can be very easy to simply attribute this to getting older.

Many of those processes, feelings, and experiences that cause us to say, "I must be getting old!" are also associated with the declining testosterone levels that occur with age. According to studies, including one published in the Journal of Clinical Endocrinology and Metabolism, symptoms associated with declining testosterone include:

- fatigue,
- lethargy,
- decreased sex drive,
- difficulty concentrating,
- mood swings,
- increased body fat, and
- decreased muscle mass.

These changes can have a substantial impact on quality of life. Looking honestly at how you've been feeling over time can help you identify some patterns you may have initially missed while busy with your daily life. Certainly, rapid changes become more obvious quickly, and we may be more likely to seek help in these cases. It's important to recognize that some changes occur more slowly but may still benefit from support.

Attending regular appointments with your healthcare providers can help you detect or confirm underlying concerns. Checking testosterone is also considered a necessary standard component of checkups for men as they age. For instance, the Mayo Clinic recommends all men over the age of fifty have testosterone levels checked once per year as a part of routine care.

These checkups help you stay ahead of the game and can be integral in your plan to prevent future health concerns. Ultimately, these provide an opportunity to further follow up on the benefits of the positive habits you build at home.

Strategies for Managing Age-Related Hormonal Changes

Whether you address concerns with medications or supplements, building positive lifestyle habits is the cornerstone of improving your health. Building healthy dietary and exercise habits improves metabolism, lowering the risk of cardiovascular disease and diabetes. These habits are also linked to improved stress management. And positive lifestyle habits are not only beneficial in these areas, but in their direct correlations with increased levels of testosterone as well.

Multiple studies have suggested different forms of exercise are associated with higher levels of testosterone in both the short and long term. For instance, a study published in the Journal of Applied Physiology found higher testosterone levels in men who performed resistance training; i.e., weight-lifting exercises. Other forms of exercise have also been beneficial—HIIT or high-intensity interval training is associated with higher testosterone levels, too (Timón 2007).

These exercises and cardiovascular training, like jogging, biking, or ellipticals, are also great ways to burn calories. If weight loss is among your goals, this is ultimately accomplished by creating a caloric deficit or burning more calories than you consume. Burning fat while building or maintaining muscle and a healthy body weight are very common goals. Creating and sticking to an exercise routine that complements your diet is the most effective way to accomplish this.

The American Dietetic Association recommends a diet high in lean protein while limiting processed foods for men over the age of fifty, but this general recommendation can be beneficial for men of all ages. This will limit sources of unhealthy fats, sugar, and excess salt. Lean protein provides the building blocks for building and maintaining muscle mass.

Diet can be a common source of pitfalls, even when you take steps to address it. If you are restricting calories, doing this without restricting nutrients can be a delicate balance. Ultimately, regardless of whether or not you are restricting calories for the purpose of losing weight, the foods you want to focus on should be nutrient-dense.

Sources of lean protein and healthy fats like salmon provide protein for muscles and healthy fats for hormone production. Whole grains, fruits, and vegetables provide fiber, improving digestion and sugar metabolism. Fruits and vegetables are also excellent sources of many crucial vitamins and minerals.

When lifestyle changes aren't enough to tip the scales in favor of healthy testosterone levels, direct hormone replacement therapy via prescription is an option for some individuals. As with any medication, the risks must be considered along with the potential benefits. When testosterone is supplemented directly, some of the risks are significant. The Urology Care Foundation recommends a thorough discussion with your healthcare provider about the potential risks, which include higher rates of heart disease and prostate cancer.

For those who prefer natural solutions, supplements are available that may help increase testosterone levels. Examples of natural products with some supporting evidence include fenugreek and D-aspartic acid. The trade-off is that these products have relatively limited studies supporting their benefit at this time. Future research may provide a clearer picture of ideal dosing, those most likely to benefit, and the degree of positive impact. Before starting any new medication or supplement, discuss the risks and benefits with a healthcare provider.

Building a Support System for the Journey

Maintaining the proper mindset is crucial. This isn't about a destination or a particular specific outcome to be achieved. Even if you successfully reach a goal, how will you stay there? It would be inadvisable to pack things up and say, "Well, I made it! I guess I'm done here." Maintaining health is about embracing the journey itself, the peaks and the valleys—and there are likely to be some valleys.

Even the most fiercely independent and self-sufficient among us can acknowledge there are some things better accomplished with the help of others. Take building a house. You could conceivably do this alone, but why in the world would you? There's wonderful pre-cut lumber to be purchased, foregoing the need to find a sufficient set of trees to chop. There are electricians that can help you get connected to the grid and wire your home, so there's a minimal risk of a fire every time you turn a light on. There are plumbers that provide access to running water and municipal sewage systems. Out of sight, out of mind. It's outstanding.

We achieve great things with community and support. You don't need to face setbacks alone, and your successes can take on additional significance when shared with others. Build your personal support system to help maintain motivation, validation, and emotional support through shared experiences. Talk about your challenges and your triumphs with family, friends, healthcare providers, or support groups. Great resources and platforms are available to find support among like-minded individuals with similar concerns, like the Men's Health Network and Hormone Health Network, among many others.

Mental health has been a complicated topic over time, but thankfully, we are learning how to be more open as a society. We all face challenges related to stress. We all feel down at times. Navigating negative feelings and emotions becomes a barrier for a large number of people. Estimates of the prevalence of anxiety and depression symptoms among adults in the United States are at about one-third of people over the last year. Some argue these rates are potentially higher due to underreporting. You are not alone in these feelings. It's also important to remember hormonal changes can make them more likely.

Reaching out and developing connections doesn't just have to be about your journey, either; it can also give you an opportunity to lend a hand to others who are struggling. You may be instrumental in someone's ability to pick up the pieces during a difficult situation and ultimately stay on track.

Chapter Seven

Navigating the Seas of Change: Understanding Andropause

Decoding Andropause: More than Just "Male Menopause"

The concept of andropause, or the male version of menopause, can be somewhat confusing. While both men and women experience age-related declines in the production of sex hormones, there are some fundamental differences. The term "pause" implies function is relatively normal until "pausing," like flipping a switch. This can be more accurately applied to the end of menstrual cycles resulting from an estrogen deficiency in females, but there are no hard endpoints to reference in men.

Instead, we see a steady decline in hormone production taking place over the course of decades. As we've seen, the decline is typically around 1 percent each year, so the decrease in testosterone can be fairly slow. The resulting symptoms can be subtle and ambiguous. They might even be missed, partially because they develop slowly and partially because they can be attributed to other concerns. These changes may have a significant impact on health and quality of life over time. Awareness of the signs and symptoms of deficiency can help you identify problems before they have a greater impact on your overall health and well-being.

Recognizing the Symptoms: More than Just a Midlife Crisis

A common theme among hormonal imbalances is the potential for a snowball effect. As one aspect of health is thrown askew, several others may follow suit. Our bodies' systems are connected. For instance, as testosterone declines, metabolism is affected. The body creates more fat stores. These fat stores alter the levels of hormones that define hunger, leading to a desire for more calories. It's a cycle; one that has the potential to contribute to higher rates of diabetes and heart disease.

Catching imbalances early can help keep small problems from growing bigger down the road. Many of the signs of hormonal imbalance can be subtle or written off as simply associated with aging or a "mid-life crisis." Some of the signs of low testosterone—fatigue, depression, irritability, decreases in muscle mass, lower bone density, and sexual dysfunction—can be easy to downplay or even miss. We may not be aware of lower bone density until a bone breaks. Having less energy is a nebulous concept that can take on different meanings for different individuals, and moving a bit more slowly is very easily attributed to aging in and of itself.

The concept of a mid-life crisis is interesting, and there is an overarching tendency to poke fun at or be dismissive of the idea. For instance, there have been stereotypical associations with sudden uncontrollable urges to buy a convertible. The humor, of course, is in the potentially irrational responses associated with coming to terms with our own mortality. As we become increasingly aware of our bodies' limitations, a broader view of life's accomplishments and our perceptions of our own identities can take shape. Ultimately, this can lead to a "crisis" of sorts, defined by an urge to make potentially significant changes.

Of course, this desire for change can drive you in a number of directions, but let's continue to consider the convertible for a moment. That convertible may be impractical, but it's *fun*. Arguably, there's a search for balance implicit in that convertible. It's a desire to breathe, feel free, and simply live in those moments where we may find respite from the mounting responsibilities of daily life. There are potentially less expensive avenues to explore the practice of mindfulness and living in the moment, but there is a worthy intent. Downplaying the way you feel stifles opportunities for personal growth.

Regardless of the cause, heightened awareness can certainly be an opportunity for positive change. It's also important to note that these changes we experience in our bodies and our mindset can also be heavily influenced and defined by hormonal changes, in addition to simple aging processes. Many of the changes we perceive can serve as a catalyst for taking more proactive steps toward maintaining health over time.

Managing Andropause: It's All in the Lifestyle

Taking steps to manage your hormonal health can lead you in a number of different directions. Upon talking with your doctor about potential concerns, if a testosterone deficit is confirmed, prescription medications may be recommended for some individuals. Regardless of whether prescriptions are considered, lifestyle is central to improving your overall health. This holds true for preventing hormonal imbalances and the associated fallout as well.

The basic tenets can be divided into a few areas and expanded on from there. Some of the most helpful areas to focus on include:

- exercise,

- diet,

- sleep, and

- stress management.

Staying active and establishing a consistent exercise routine has a multitude of benefits, ranging from broad to specific associations with hormonal health. Of course, there are the metabolic benefits. You're burning calories, preventing excess fat build-up, controlling cholesterol, and keeping your metabolism humming. There are direct benefits for your heart, improving its ability to pump oxygen throughout the body efficiently and lowering the risk of heart attack and stroke. The idea of "if you're not using it, you're losing it" is often associated with muscle mass but also holds true for bone density. When you keep moving, your bones and joints benefit as well.

Establishing a routine helps, and activities as simple as walking are beneficial. Some exercise routines have the potential to be more impactful, however, and studies directly relate increased testosterone levels with these exercises. A study published in the Journal of Applied Physiology suggests strength training—i.e., resistance or weight training—is directly associated with higher testosterone levels. High-intensity interval training (HIIT) has also been associated directly with higher levels of testosterone (Timón 2007). These exercises involve alternating between periods of relative rest and explosive exertion. They may not be appropriate for everyone, but they can be an excellent way to burn calories and trim fat. If you're unsure how to implement these exercises safely, be sure to talk with a personal trainer or other healthcare provider.

Maintaining a healthy diet is also highly beneficial. Your diet can be leveraged to work for you, providing all of the essential vitamins, minerals, and building blocks needed to support healthy hormone production. Balanced sources of lean proteins, healthy fats, whole grains, fruits, and vegetables provide the nutrients you need to keep moving and feel great. Hormonal production, along with many other processes in the body, can operate at a high level when you eat well.

Just as your body benefits from activity and a healthy diet, it also needs rest. The National Sleep Foundation recommends sleeping between seven to nine hours each night. This time is crucial, as it allows our bodies to repair cells and restore energy.

Sleep also influences and is influenced by hormone production cycles. One of the more prominent daily hormonal cycles associated with sleep is that of cortisol. This hormone, among others, plays a role in keeping us active and alert. Increased levels are also associated with stress and feeling tense or ready to move. Over the course of the day, cortisol levels dwindle and eventually reach a point conducive to rest before peaking again at the start of the next day. A lack of sleep disrupts this cycle. Higher levels of cortisol ultimately open the door to other imbalances, including testosterone.

Of course, when we're stressed, sleep can be harder to come by. This is partly due to continued cortisol elevations lasting into the evening, making it difficult for your body to get the rest it needs. Stress is a common component of daily life, and while finding ways to reduce your sources of stress can be beneficial, it may not always be practical. Stressors are likely to be there, and building a toolkit to help manage their impact is vital to maintaining balance.

Remember, there's potential for a cascading effect when stress isn't managed and cortisol runs rampant. Using tools such as mindfulness meditation and deep (diaphragmatic) breathing has been shown to directly lower cortisol levels. In turn, testosterone production is able to continue relatively unhindered.

Seeking Medical Help: When to Reach Out

Enacting lifestyle changes and continuing a healthy lifestyle is the foundation of maintaining a healthy hormonal balance. Whether existing problems have been identified or you're seeking to prevent health concerns, diet, exercise, and stress management are always important. There are times when these steps aren't enough, however, and it's crucial to be able to recognize when further help is needed.

When symptoms persist—especially if they impact your quality of life—it's time to reach out to a healthcare provider. This should be done in addition to regular, routine checkups throughout andropause. These checkups allow for establishing baselines, identifying changes over time, and finding and addressing potential problems before they have a greater impact. As testosterone declines, the risks of cardiovascular disease, osteoporosis, and mood disorders increase.

In some instances, direct testosterone replacement therapy may be considered. These treatments can have a considerable positive impact, but it's very important to have a thorough conversation with a healthcare provider about potential risks and side effects. For instance, testosterone replacement therapy (TRT) can ultimately increase the risk of cardiovascular disease and may contribute to a heightened risk of certain types of cancer. These factors should be considered carefully when establishing a plan for protecting overall health.

Keeping open communication with your healthcare providers allows you to monitor your progress more completely. Ultimately, we want to make sure our efforts are effective. These checkups allow for identifying real, quantifiable improvements and maintaining stability.

Andropause and Mental Health: an Often-Overlooked Connection

Over the years, some troubling trends have been established. The National Institute of Mental Health states men have been less likely to recognize, talk openly about, and seek help for symptoms of depression. The same holds true for symptoms of anxiety. This may ultimately be a cultural phenomenon defined by a fear of judgment or a negative stigma.

Stoicism plays well in the movies, but it doesn't always translate well to real life. Acknowledging and taking steps to address challenges, whatever they may be, takes strength and courage. Appearing "tough" and being mentally and emotionally strong are two very different things.

Professional athletes are excellent examples of this. Football is a mainstay, if you turn on the television on a Sunday afternoon in autumn and into the winter. At first glance, the NFL appears to be a bastion of toughness, where weakness is quickly weeded out, and only the strongest can be depended on to deliver consistently and develop a career with meaningful longevity. What may not be readily apparent is that mental strength and physical strength are equally important, and these athletes take this to heart.

There are team psychologists offering forms of cognitive behavioral therapy (CBT). Players practice mindfulness, limiting negative self-talk and building the focus needed to compete at the highest level. Quarterbacks like Kirk Cousins employ biofeedback techniques to increase the mind-body connection. These practices are also closely related to and considered core components of meditation. Making split decisions requires clarity, and this clarity is often achieved with help. Prioritizing mental health is vital to many measures of success, even among those role models famous for their toughness.

On a personal level, changing the conversation about mental health may not be as important as simply having it in the first place. Giving yourself grace is important, as well as knowing that the challenges you face are not unique—they are shared by many. Talking about it and taking steps to manage these challenges is not a weakness and can only make you stronger.

It's also important to remember that the changes associated with andropause lead to fatigue, irritability, and a higher likelihood of experiencing symptoms of depression and anxiety. This is chemistry, not a personal shortcoming. However, you can do something about these potential changes when you're aware of them.

Many resources are available; perhaps the most important being family and friends. Staying open, building your own support structure, and becoming a part of others' support networks is tremendously helpful. Stay connected.

There are also healthcare resources available, including therapy services. Cognitive behavior therapy extends beyond simply talking—it's a structured approach provided by an experienced professional to help you identify patterns in your thinking and implement personalized strategies to manage negative thoughts and emotions. Therapy sessions can be very effective, helping you build a skillset that serves you well over the long term.

Medications are also often prescribed and can be used either in combination with therapy or alone, depending on personal preferences. Each therapeutic option comes with its own set of benefits and potential risks, all of which are best discussed with a provider on an individual basis. The first step is recognizing patterns that may be of concern or accepting feedback from those close to you. Even if you ultimately do not have a diagnosable condition, talking openly about your concerns opens the door for fresh perspectives and new paths forward.

Chapter Eight

Decoding Hormone Test Results: Your Personal Guide

Understanding Your Hormone Tests

You've spoken with your doctor, and tests have been ordered. Hormone levels are among those being assessed, and you wonder, "What do these results mean?" Let's take some time to review some basics before diving into more detail and ultimately discussing what you can *do* with these results.

Hormone levels can be tested in several ways, including blood tests or measurements in urine or saliva. Ranges considered normal are provided alongside your results, and you should have a chance to discuss the results with your provider. A common complaint is the potential for a relatively brief explanation during or after a clinic visit, which is why it's helpful to be armed with some knowledge of your own to provide context and guide questions that may be more helpful to you.

Using statistics, reference ranges provide a sense of what could be considered "normal" across a population. The ranges vary depending on the type of test being used, along with individual factors, like age and the presence of any other health concerns. It's important to give your healthcare provider context by providing an accurate medical history. There are a number of health concerns that can contribute to testosterone decline, like low thyroid function, obesity, difficulty sleeping, and other chronic illnesses. Good communication allows for individualized care.

It's important to remember that these test results represent a snapshot in time. The hormone levels in our bodies are constantly changing, including predictable peaks and valleys over the course of each day. Cortisol is highest in the morning and fades throughout the day. Testosterone follows a similar pattern. Your tests will likely be ordered for a specific time with these fluctuations in mind, so it's important to follow the instructions for the test.

Making Sense of Testosterone Levels

Testosterone usually takes center stage for men among hormone test results, as it's a key player in many areas of men's health. Reference ranges can vary between labs, which has been a point of contention among clinicians. Ultimately, the American Urological Association has provided guidelines referencing serum (blood) total testosterone levels of less than 300 ng/dL as partially indicative of a clinical testosterone deficiency. The term *partially* is used because a second, confirming lab test is needed, along with the presence of symptoms related to testosterone deficiency.

A potential source of confusion is the expert panel's agreement on a range of 450–600 ng/dL being considered a normal physiologic range. The low end of normal is significantly higher than the level deemed a clinical deficiency. Ultimately, test results in the 300–450 ng/dL range are up to the patient and provider's discretion and may result in recommendations for lifestyle modifications. If clinical treatment is started, reaching levels greater than 450 ng/dL becomes a common target.

It's important to communicate any symptoms you may be experiencing, especially if they aren't readily apparent in a physical examination. Symptoms associated with low testosterone that are important to mention include:

- fatigue,

- lower motivation or work/physical performance,

- poor concentration,

- impaired memory,

- vision changes,

- reduced sex drive or erectile dysfunction,

- changes in mood; i.e., irritability, depression, or anxiety, and

- changes in muscle mass.

Abnormally high levels of testosterone are fairly rare but can result in a higher risk of cardiovascular disease, aggressive behavior, and certain types of cancer. If a healthcare provider is concerned your testosterone levels are too high, it's likely further testing will be recommended to identify the cause.

It's important to note that hormone test results often provide two different numbers related to testosterone. These are total testosterone and free testosterone. Total testosterone is a measure of all the testosterone in the blood, including the free, unbound testosterone and the testosterone bound to proteins like sex hormone-binding globulin (SHBG). Free testosterone is unbound and free to exert the effects of testosterone throughout the body. Typically, free testosterone is available at a ratio of about 1 to 2 percent of total testosterone, but the availability of proteins like SHBG can alter this ratio. Both total and free testosterone are important measures. Free testosterone predicts hormonal activity by measuring active testosterone and can provide a window into overall hormonal health. However, total testosterone has been used more frequently throughout the years in clinical diagnosis and treatment guidelines.

Interpreting Other Hormone Levels

While monitoring testosterone levels is important, test results are also likely to include the levels of other hormones in the body. These often include cortisol, estrogen, and thyroid hormones. Each of these plays a role in many of the same functions within the body that testosterone does, or can influence testosterone production. It's important to understand how these hormones affect the overall picture.

Cortisol is most closely associated with stress. As levels rise, we become more alert, and as levels fall, we are more able to rest. Increased levels are strongly associated with a sympathetic nervous response, or the muscle tension and rapid heart rate associated with stress and anxiety. Cortisol influences how the body uses its resources, including producing other hormones. When cortisol levels are high, testosterone production can slow down in favor of other processes.

Estrogen plays an integral role in maintaining healthy bones and sexual function in men, but a balance is needed. When levels become higher, men can experience symptoms like breast enlargement (gynecomastia) and fertility concerns due to reduced sperm production. Some medications, stress, diet, and liver conditions can cause relatively higher estrogen levels, and higher body fat percentages predict higher rates of conversion of testosterone to estrogen in the body.

Thyroid hormones are instrumental in defining metabolism. Lower thyroid levels are associated with fatigue, lower energy levels, and increased body weight and fat stores. These changes in metabolic rate and body composition can influence the circulating levels of sex hormones. As body fat rises, we also see an associated rise in the rate of conversion of testosterone to estrogen.

There is a connection between TSH, or thyroid-stimulating hormone, and cortisol, as well. TSH is responsible for promoting the release of thyroid hormones—when the body perceives thyroid levels as being too low, TSH levels rise. Elevated TSH levels have also been associated with higher cortisol levels, leading to the potential for further imbalance.

These hormones, among many others, work closely together in an often delicate balance. When the levels of one hormone are higher or lower, this can cause others to be thrown askew. Reviewing these results with a healthcare provider can help you take a step back and see the full picture, identifying those areas that may be most helpful to address to improve your health moving forward.

Using Your Test Results to Improve Your Health

With your hormone test results in hand, you now have another piece of the puzzle to help you define your current health. Armed with a greater understanding of how your lifestyle can impact hormone levels and how these hormones impact overall health, you can begin to define areas of your health that are likely to benefit the most from making adjustments.

If testosterone levels are low, this can provide either a direct or partial explanation for troublesome symptoms. There are ways to support healthy testosterone production, like improving your diet, getting adequate exercise, and taking steps to manage stress. Focusing on each of these areas is helpful for maintaining existing balance.

If cortisol levels are high, you know stress management may be particularly important for achieving balance. Find ways to incorporate deep breathing techniques, mindfulness, or meditation because each of these is associated with significant drops in cortisol. These techniques can also be combined with exercise by practicing yoga, making it an excellent way to promote overall wellness.

Remember, hormone test results are a snapshot. You may be able to infer some ideas about general trends, but testing regularly will give you a much more precise picture of the changes occurring over time. If you've made changes in your lifestyle, or have begun using a supplement or medication, followup testing allows you to see the impact those changes have had. Is what you're doing working? Are there adjustments that could be made?

Track results over time, along with the changes you've made and the frequency and severity of symptoms you experience. The benefits are twofold. Of course, this allows for identifying trends and correlations over time as you monitor to ensure improvements and validation of your efforts. It also helps you become more accustomed to listening to your body, which is a skill that can be developed. As daily life marches on, our minds are often elsewhere. Paying attention to your body and its signals is a process improved by meaningful intent.

It's also important to remember that hormone tests are useful, but they are one piece of a larger puzzle. Health must be considered holistically, and establishing a relationship with and consistently discussing your results and status with a trusted healthcare provider can help you keep the larger picture in focus.

There can be times when hormone test results are slightly out of a normal range but you're feeling fine. Positive lifestyle changes are never a bad idea, but a lack of symptoms leads to fewer immediate concerns related to the results. This is especially true if only one test remains out of range and others are normal—something you would not be aware of without consistent testing.

On the other hand, you may have symptoms that concern you, but your results return completely normal. In these cases, it's time to dig deeper and explore other potential causes with your provider. In either of these scenarios, you now have valuable information to help you move forward.

Next Steps after Your Hormone Test

Remembering that your test results are a snapshot representing one point in time is an important concept. When devoid of context, these results are ultimately meaningless for several reasons. The symptoms you experience (or a lack thereof), the potential contributing factors like other chronic conditions, and developing a sense of the direction and rate of change at which your levels are moving are all important. Speaking with your healthcare provider can help you combine these pieces and develop a well-informed plan.

If your hormone levels require support, recommendations can often include lifestyle changes, medications, or hormone replacement therapy (HRT). Medications, supplements, HRT, and even some lifestyle changes are not devoid of risk. It's always best to have a thorough conversation with your healthcare provider about your options and find the best path to promote your overall health.

Whether broadly cultural or fueled by a desire for simplicity, a tendency is to depend on treatments for a fix. Regardless of whether you're ultimately using injectable HRT or natural supplements, positive lifestyle changes are central to the success of any therapeutic approach. The effects of a healthy diet, consistent exercise, and practicing good sleep hygiene can be substantial—in some cases, these changes may be all you need. Great places to start include cutting back on processed foods and sources of sugar, making stress-reduction skills and activities a priority, and establishing healthy sleep habits.

Regular follow-ups with your provider and routine testing aren't the only useful tools for assessing your initial status and developing a plan. They also help you monitor the successes and any shortfalls of a plan you've brought into action. These help you adjust, make improvements when needed, and validate the positive impact of your efforts. The recommended frequency of testing can vary depending on individual factors. Regardless of how often your healthcare providers suggest you test over time, it's helpful to track these results yourself, along with making notes about changes in your approach and any symptoms you experience.

Chapter Nine

Weighing the Pros and Cons of Hormone Replacement Therapy

Understanding Hormone Replacement Therapy

The term hormone replacement therapy (HRT) is most often associated with menopause. A quick search online reveals an abundance of information about estrogen and progesterone treatments, and hardly any about testosterone. For this reason, the term may lead to some potential confusion, but it can also be extended to testosterone. Testosterone is indeed a hormone in need of replacement in some circumstances. It's important to recognize the areas in which it's most likely to help—and what some of the limitations may be. In current research, testosterone has been associated with improvements in:

- erectile dysfunction,
- libido,
- anemia,
- bone density (and potentially fracture risk, although a direct connection is less clear),
- lean body mass, and
- depressive symptoms.

Current research has ultimately been inconclusive when evaluating testosterone for improvements in:

- cognitive function,
- energy,
- cholesterol levels,
- blood sugar control, and
- overall quality of life.

There are significant risks associated with therapy, so it's important to be aware of where the benefits lie and weigh them against those risks based on individual needs.

For those who have consulted their physician, had their testosterone levels checked (likely at least twice), and determined replacement therapy is needed, there are a variety of dosage forms available. These include skin patches, gels, injections, and implants, and each comes with its own individual pros and cons. Once optimal dosage is established, the effects of testosterone in systemic circulation are largely the same. The primary differences lie in the frequency of administration and the potential for local discomfort, so the choice often comes down to personal preference. Let's take some time to explore these options.

Testosterone injections have traditionally been used intramuscularly, but there are increasing numbers of patients and clinicians who opt for a subcutaneous route (under the skin). Of course, there is the potential for injection site pain and localized muscle pain from the needle itself and the introduction of fluid volume into the tissue. This varies little when compared with vaccines and other injectables. If you don't mind other injections, it's unlikely testosterone injections would present unique issues with the injection itself.

Testosterone injections are available in several forms, with their differences characterized primarily by how long they remain active after injection. This will translate directly into how often you'd need to inject them to reach a steady state. The options available are:

- Testosterone cypionate: longer-acting, injected once every one to four weeks.

- Testosterone enanthate: intermediate, injected one to two times weekly.

- Testosterone propionate: shorter-acting, injected once every two to three days.

- Testosterone undecanoate: significantly longer-acting, injected every twelve weeks by a healthcare professional.

Individual needs and response to therapy define the dose and frequency during follow-up.

Topical gels provide another option for testosterone delivery, with several potential routes of administration. Natesto is formulated specifically for application in the nostrils and is absorbed through the nasal mucosa. Systemic effects are similar overall, and the product has a higher incidence of local side effects—like nosebleeds, or a runny or stuffy nose—and potential changes in smell.

Other gels include Androgel, Testim, and Fortesta, each of which is commonly applied to the shoulders or upper arms but may also be applied to the abdomen. Local skin reactions like itching and rash are potential side effects unique to these formulations. It's crucial to note that the medication can be transferred through touch, which can cause significant side effects in women and children. If you are using a gel form of testosterone, it's best to let the area dry completely before physical contact with others (be mindful of transfer to your own clothing as well).

Androderm patches provide a similar approach, delivering testosterone through a patch continuously over time. Local skin reactions, including those related to adhesives, are possible when using patches.

Striant provides testosterone via a tablet that adheres to the gum once inserted in the mouth. Testosterone is released and absorbed through the oral mucosa. Similar to other delivery methods, unique local side effects, such as gum or mouth irritation and bitter taste, are more likely.

Testopel offers testosterone in the form of a small pellet that is implanted under the skin, usually near the hip or buttocks. These offer a slow, steady release of testosterone over the course of several months. Monitoring the injection site for pain and swelling after the implant is placed is important.

Some prescription medications are also employed that promote testosterone production in the body rather than replacing it directly. Clomiphene (Clomid) is an example of this, as it stimulates testosterone production through its effects on the pituitary gland. In men, the benefits of clomiphene must be weighed against the potential impact on cardiovascular risk and liver function, among other possible side effects.

Human chorionic gonadotropin (hCG) is used in some instances. Its activity promotes increased testosterone production in the testes. It can be paired with other methods of testosterone replacement if deemed appropriate by a healthcare professional.

Among each of these methods, systemic effects are largely the same. Deciding on a therapeutic approach ultimately relies on carefully considering the benefits and ensuring they outweigh the risks for each individual's unique circumstances. Improvements in sexual dysfunction, energy, and mood can have a substantial positive impact on quality of life. However, it's important to consider risks carefully to ensure a fully informed decision.

Risks Associated with Hormone Replacement Therapy

Armed with the knowledge of the symptoms most likely to improve with testosterone therapy, a sense of the delivery options, and the risks associated with each of those options, it's time to look more generally at the risks of hormone replacement therapy. If you've spent much time researching testosterone replacement therapy online or have spoken with family or friends, you may have come across a number of potential side effects and risks. It's helpful to take some time to break these down, so you can gain a sense of how they may affect you directly.

First and foremost, there are the immediately apparent potential side effects. Many of these can be bothersome but may not be considered outright dangerous in their own right. Some of these are specific to the form of delivery, like injection site pain. Other side effects include things like:

- acne,

- labored breathing while sleeping,

- breast swelling and tenderness, and

- swelling in the feet and ankles

These side effects can be managed or reversed if therapy is stopped. Stopping may not be a simple process, however.

It's helpful to keep in mind that the body becomes somewhat reliant on an outside source of testosterone once it's introduced consistently. The testosterone production occurring in your body slows down considerably, partially due to a feedback loop in which your body responds to the presence of circulating testosterone by stopping its own production—it's already there, so you must not need more. Testicular production drops and the testicles themselves can shrink.

If therapy is stopped, levels drop, and it takes time for your natural production to rebound. While there's not necessarily a withdrawal in the sense we may be most familiar with (i.e., opioids.), symptoms of low testosterone return, potentially more pronounced than previously experienced, and a form of dependence can be established.

A potentially higher risk of developing blood clots is a much more serious concern and becomes a focus of monitoring as therapy continues. Testosterone therapy is an effective means of preventing anemia as red blood cell production is stimulated. Unfortunately, though, if red blood cell counts become too high, this can lead to a higher risk of clotting.

Broader concerns have also been raised related to elevated risks of cardiovascular disease and prostate cancer. Studies have ultimately been mixed related to prostate cancer, and the relatively short-term nature of existing studies has made a causative relationship difficult to establish. If you are at risk of developing prostate cancer, this potential association may be a cause for significant concern.

In 2010, a prominent study called the Testosterone in Older Men study was stopped early because individuals receiving testosterone had significantly more heart problems. This raised concerns related to the potential for an increased risk of cardiovascular events like heart attacks, strokes, and heart-related deaths.

More recent reviews have questioned whether these risks can or should be extended to younger populations. Younger age groups have not seen the same significant increase in cardiovascular events, but again, trial periods were relatively short. The effects of elevated risks may have a more immediate impact on an aging population. Ultimately, especially if you have existing cardiovascular risk factors or a history of cardiovascular disease, the potential for further elevating your risk could be significant.

If you're considering testosterone replacement therapy, these are important factors to discuss with your healthcare provider. This offers an opportunity to dive deeper into your own individual benefits and risks and determine whether treatment may be right for you.

Natural Alternatives to Hormone Replacement Therapy

Weighing the potential risks and benefits of testosterone replacement therapy can feel daunting, and that's okay. It's good to take the time to think things through and explore all your options. For some, taking a more natural approach may be more comfortable. As we discussed earlier in the nutrition and herbal supplements sections, there are several natural ways to support hormone balance. Building on that foundation, we will take a deeper dive here into some of the nutrients and herbal supplements that can make a difference to testosterone levels.

Regardless of whether you decide to use prescription medications, taking steps to improve or maintain a healthy lifestyle is recommended and can make a significant impact in its own right. Getting consistent exercise, eating a balanced diet, and prioritizing your sleep hygiene can have a very positive impact on hormonal balance.

Many men also turn to dietary or herbal supplements for additional support. Supplements like fenugreek and ashwagandha have been associated with increased testosterone levels, which may significantly impact some individuals. It's important to bear in mind, however, that much of the research related to these supplements is limited by small sample sizes and populations that may not be representative of those most likely to have an existing testosterone deficiency (i.e., young, healthy men).

Ultimately, medical intervention may be needed, and it's best to consult a healthcare provider or a specialist who can help you devise an individualized treatment plan. In some cases, natural supplements may fit nicely with a recommended approach, and it's helpful to learn more about your options.

We'll start with nutrients that can be provided by your diet or supplemented with over-the-counter products. These can help establish the building blocks that support healthy testosterone production.

Vitamin D is critical for overall health, including mood, cardiovascular health, and testosterone production. Getting outside in the sun helps your body produce this naturally, but it can be difficult to make enough if you're living in a climate plagued by winter. Fortunately, supplements are available, and vitamin D is also found in fatty fish and fortified foods like milk.

Due to effective marketing during cold and flu season, zinc is often synonymous with a healthy immune system. It's also a critical component of many proteins and enzymes that act as catalysts for a variety of other bodily functions, including testosterone synthesis. Zinc is found in nutritional supplements and foods like oysters, beef, pumpkin seeds, and cashews.

Vitamin B6 supports brain health, energy levels, and red blood cell production while also helping to regulate steroid hormone levels. It's sometimes listed as pyridoxine and can be found in supplements like B complex or standalone products. It's also present in poultry, fish, and bananas. Vitamin B12 supports energy levels as well and is found in meat products, fish, dairy, and certain fortified foods.

Magnesium, like zinc, is a mineral that plays a role in testosterone synthesis. It may also promote healthy sleep, which is critical for establishing and maintaining hormonal balance. Nuts, seeds, leafy greens, and whole grains all provide dietary sources of magnesium. If you take a magnesium supplement, it's important to be aware that it's a laxative at higher doses. If your stools become loose, consider holding the dose for a day or two and then lowering it.

Omega-3 fatty acids are healthy fats. They can provide benefits for heart health, may have anti-inflammatory effects, and act as important precursors to testosterone during natural production. Fatty fish, avocados, flaxseeds, and walnuts are excellent sources of omega-3.

These are all critical nutrients, and deficiencies lead to a variety of health concerns. Poor production of testosterone is one of the many ways nutritional deficiencies can impact your health.

Herbal supplements are also popular and may arguably provide a more targeted approach that extends beyond generalized support. These have more limited clinical evidence supporting their use but have, in some cases, been used for centuries (or longer) in various forms of traditional medicine. However, it's important to keep in mind that the potential risks can be just as poorly documented as the potential benefits, and these supplements can interact with existing medications and health conditions.

As we saw earlier, ashwagandha is among the herbal supplements with the most clinical support. As an adaptogenic herb, it has been seen to reduce cortisol levels, and several studies have suggested testosterone levels may be increased directly by ashwagandha as well. Overall, the sample sizes of studies are fairly small, however, and the doses and forms of ashwagandha provided to participants aren't standardized (some provide root preparations, some provide leaf preparations, and others are extracts produced by various means), so it can be difficult to predict a consistent response across a general population.

Fenugreek also has some clinical support for directly raising testosterone levels and libido. Similar to ashwagandha, it's difficult to extend a predictive effect to a general population, but current research holds some promise. While generally well tolerated, there have been some potential concerns related to low blood sugars when taken in high doses by individuals managing diabetes. Care should be taken by these individuals before adding fenugreek to a medication regimen.

Tongkat Ali (*Eurycoma longifolia*) has long been used in Southeast Asian traditional medicine for a variety of purposes, including treating malaria, infections, male infertility, and erectile dysfunction. In clinical studies, results have been promising and do show an associated rise in testosterone levels. One more targeted trial has also been conducted, suggesting a potential benefit for erectile dysfunction in aging men.

Further research would be beneficial, but the existing research provides some backing to the traditional consideration of Tongkat Ali as an aphrodisiac.

Ginger has shown some preliminary promise related to testosterone production. It may help boost testosterone levels through mechanisms like antioxidant activity and improved cholesterol availability in the testes, which acts as a precursor in testosterone synthesis. It's important to note that ginger is not recommended for individuals taking blood thinners, as it can increase the risk of bleeding.

Dehydroepiandrosterone, or DHEA, is a hormone that acts as a precursor to testosterone. Like testosterone, levels of DHEA decline over time as we age. DHEA supplements have been associated with some positive effects on testosterone levels and erectile function, but it's important to be mindful of risks. There are some concerns related to the potential for DHEA supplementation to cause increased rates of prostate cancer. DHEA is also a precursor for estrogen, which can lead to side effects like gynecomastia (breast enlargement) and hair loss.

Pine pollen provides a source of phytoandrogens. Androgens are, of course, sex hormones, including testosterone. *Phyto* refers to a plant origin, so the term phytoandrogen refers to androgens derived from plants. Phytoandrogens are structurally similar to testosterone and could theoretically have similar activity in the body (this has also been proposed as a potential approach to managing BPH or an enlarged prostate). The effects, both positive and potentially negative, have not been studied extensively in humans, however.

Nettle root has been suggested for use in managing an enlarged prostate, and during some trials, an increase in serum testosterone has also been observed. It has been proposed that nettle root accomplishes this by preventing the breakdown of testosterone, allowing levels to begin to build up. Clinical research is ultimately limited, however, leaving some open-ended questions related to its safety and efficacy across broad populations.

If you peruse the shelves at a local store or search online for nutritional supplements, there will be no shortage of options promising to boost your vitality and make you feel like you're eighteen years old again. Take the time to step back and evaluate the ingredients (particularly if you're looking at a product with eighteen active ingredients). Review the product with your healthcare provider to ensure there are no conflicts with any existing therapy and that the product will align with your needs and goals. Supplements can and do provide benefits to some individuals, but it's crucial to make your decisions with due diligence.

Making an Informed Decision

There is some interesting psychology associated with making decisions. Of course, we all want results. If those results can be realized sooner, that's outstanding. Once a problem is faced, there can be a sense of urgency to fix it. Of course, we can all agree that, in general, things shouldn't be rushed, but realizing we may be rushing can be difficult. After all, obligations in our daily lives can pile up, and we become conditioned to "move quickly and get things done." People who can do this efficiently are often praised for it.

The problem lies in our potential tendency never to be fully present when moving from one solution to the next. When we're constantly moving, it can be difficult to give our full attention to any particular problem or decision we're presented with. This is problematic when faced with decisions that are more complex and whose effects can be more subtle or delayed. Prioritizing or distinguishing between those times when it may be best to take a step back and give something your full attention doesn't always come naturally. This can require a conscious effort in and of itself. Moving quickly can be a difficult habit to break. Not all decisions are created equal in terms of their potential impact, but those that affect your long-term health could be considered among the most impactful.

Just as the symptoms associated with low testosterone can be life-altering in many ways, so can the treatments. Of course, the changes can be positive, but there are also potential drawbacks, and learning about these helps you weigh your choices more accurately. You wouldn't marry someone you've just met—you want to take the time to get to know them first. Similarly, taking the time to get to know your treatment options puts you in a position to be more successful in managing your health, which can change your life.

Any type of therapy to increase testosterone levels will have some benefits, carry certain risks, and have available alternatives, each with its own set of benefits and risks. Your overall past and current health affect the way you may respond to each of these options as an individual. For instance, if you have a family history of prostate cancer, your own risk of developing cancer while using testosterone replacement therapy may be increased.

Talking with your healthcare provider can provide valuable context and help to ensure that your treatment plan is the right one for you. Once you have a plan in place, it's critical to continue attending regular checkups. This gives you and your provider more information about direct measures of treatment—like hormone levels themselves and other pertinent labs—trends in your symptoms, and any potential side effects. If you start testosterone therapy, it's also crucial to have regular prostate exams to monitor for concerning changes.

Take the time to give your treatment plan your full attention. Learn about your current status and the options in front of you, and move forward with the confidence that you've made the best decision for you.

Chapter Ten

Planning for Long-term Hormonal Balance

"*A goal without a plan is just a wish.*"
- Antoine de Saint-Exupéry, French writer, poet, and pioneering aviator.

The Road to Lifelong Hormonal Balance

There is a fear associated with aging. There's an inevitability, perhaps a sense of helplessness, a worry that we may become less effective, less useful, or irrelevant. Potential societal reinforcements of these ideas exist—for instance, ageism in the workplace or the fear of having more difficulty finding work—which can leave us feeling marginalized. While some negative feedback may indeed be there, it's important to recognize that many of these thoughts are internal. An element of self-defeat can become somewhat ingrained.

Dr. Becca Levy, a prominent researcher on longevity and aging, has described visiting Japan and becoming intrigued by lifespans that are among the longest in the world. What could be contributing to this? What factors allow people to not only live longer but also live *well* longer? Naturally, our thoughts may turn to factors like gender, socioeconomic status, or loneliness. Dr. Levy noticed that there seemed to be something else at play, however—a tendency for more positive self-perceptions associated with aging. These individuals associated their own age with terms like *vital* and *wise*.

When this concept was put to the test, the results were striking. People with positive self-perceptions related to aging may live, on average, for about seven and a half years longer. Mindset is critical, and it may literally translate into a longer, more fulfilling life. Of course, a sense of intrinsic value can lead to consistent, sustained, positive lifestyle choices. Your mindset is the foundation for eating well, staying active, and taking care of yourself over time.

Ultimately, consistency over time is what's needed. Managing any aspect of your health, including hormonal health, is not achieved overnight. It's also important to remember that success is often defined more by our response to setbacks than by our ability to keep things running smoothly at all times. The road is likely to be bumpy—we all have those times when things get away from us. Eating habits may take a turn for the worse, or exercise habits may fall by the wayside. Taking steps to improve aspects of our health like diet, physical activity, and sleep may not always lead to immediately obvious benefits day to day, but the effects do add up and can have a profound impact over time.

A potentially tricky aspect of promoting long-term health benefits is related to the nature of prevention. When goals are defined by the *absence* of an event (e.g., avoiding a heart attack), it becomes simpler to define failure rather than achievement. Goals are often best set when they are clearly defined, realistic, and broken up into increments. For example, "I will replace an afternoon bag of potato chips with a handful of almonds every day this week," or, "I will walk a mile three days this week." These goals can also be extended into longer increments to build upon success: "I will reach my weekly exercise goals every week this month."

These are goals that allow for a clearly defined plan—and a sense of accomplishment. It's far easier to imagine yourself celebrating a month of good exercise habits rather than a month without suffering a stroke. In truth, however, you *have* taken steps to lower your risk. Incremental goals also allow for more immediate focus, making it easier to get back up when you stumble. If you've had a rough week, it doesn't mean your year is ruined. Next week can be better.

Numerous studies show that consistent healthy eating habits, physical activity, sleep, and stress management are all deeply beneficial for hormonal balance and overall health. Healthy choices lower the risk of cardiovascular disease, prostate disease, and sexual dysfunction, among many other health concerns. Your mindset and commitment to getting back on the path when you stumble can help you age well rather than simply age.

Tackling the Potential Health Risks of Hormone Imbalances

There can be a tendency to only focus on certain aspects of men's hormonal health, like the potential loss of muscle mass or sexual dysfunction, but it's important to recognize the impact runs much deeper. Hormones are integral to many systems in the body, and a healthy balance goes hand in hand with overall health. Testosterone alone is associated with changes in mood, energy, and the risk of developing conditions like osteoporosis and heart disease. The impact of testosterone balance is well-established in clinical literature. Research in prominent journals like the Journal of Clinical Endocrinology & Metabolism, along with national organizations like the American Heart Association, highlight the importance of testosterone directly.

Eating well, staying active, and making healthy choices have a significant impact over time. Establishing realistic goals backed by a plan can help build consistency in the long term. It can also be helpful to approach these goals with both long- and short-term increments, allowing for adjustments when life inevitably throws you a curveball. In time, healthy choices add up, promoting lower risks of hormonal imbalance and disease.

Taking steps as simple as reducing processed foods can help reduce the risk of developing metabolic imbalances leading to weight gain, insulin resistance, and type 2 diabetes. By lowering your risk of diabetes or taking steps to better manage existing concerns, you are ultimately lowering your risk of heart attack and stroke, kidney and liver damage, changes in vision, difficulty fighting infections, and nerve damage. Remember, processes in the body are heavily interconnected, and hormones are an instrumental part of these connections. Lowering the risk of metabolic imbalances can also lower the risk of developing testosterone imbalances.

Simply eating fewer processed foods and removing harmful substances can help, but it's also helpful to recognize your diet for its potential benefits. There are an abundance of vitamins, minerals, and nutrients to be leveraged. A balanced diet with lean sources of protein, whole grains, fruits, and vegetables provides the building blocks needed to promote the healthy production of hormones. This, along with adequate physical activity, sleep, and stress management make up the foundation of maintaining your health.

Even those with the most consistent healthy lifestyle habits benefit from monitoring hormone levels over time. While imbalance can be made less likely to occur, the potential for low testosterone still exists. This is why it's important to regularly attend appointments with your healthcare providers. Labs can give you a direct sense of current status, and regularly keeping appointments can reveal trends over time. When concerns are caught early, they are simpler to address before they develop into much larger, more impactful health problems.

Maintaining Hormonal Balance with Age

As we age, our bodies naturally undergo changes. Hormone production, including testosterone, tends to decrease as we age. However, just because these changes occur doesn't mean we must accept declining health as inevitable.

Research from prominent organizations, like the National Institute on Aging, and experts, such as those at the Mayo Clinic, agrees that maintaining healthy lifestyle choices makes a substantial difference for those seeking to maintain optimal hormone levels and health. Research consistently points to primary factors like physical activity, balanced diet, and healthy sleep patterns, associating these with maintained hormonal balance over the years.

Prevention is the best medicine. In addition to attending regular screenings and appointments with healthcare providers, it's helpful to keep healthy choices in mind on a day-to-day basis. Choose whole foods over processed options, get outside for some fresh air and exercise, and establish a bedtime routine that consistently promotes the sleep you need to thrive.

The importance of sleep cannot be overstated. It is critical for hormonal balance and overall health. The National Sleep Foundation highlights associations with adequate sleep, longer life spans, and higher quality of life. If this has been something you've struggled with, it can be tremendously helpful to seek additional help. Medications can be beneficial, but there are many ways to find support. This includes targeted cognitive behavioral therapy with individuals who specialize in providing insomnia management techniques. Your body needs this rest to recharge and keep producing the hormones that help you maintain a healthy balance.

Studies have also shown that regular exercise, like strength or resistance training and aerobic exercise, can upregulate testosterone production. Some of this also appears to be increased amounts of testosterone converted from DHEA in local muscle tissue when muscles are activated. So we see that establishing exercise routines can not only build and maintain muscle, it can build and maintain testosterone, as well. This, in turn, becomes a positive chemical factor for maintaining muscle and bone mass in and of itself.

Here are ten recommended exercises specifically targeting men's hormone health that not only help tone your physique but also boost hormone health:

1. Squats:

    - target large muscle groups, stimulating testosterone and growth hormone release, and

    - improve overall lower body strength and muscle mass.

2. Deadlifts:

    ◦ engage multiple muscle groups, promoting testosterone production, and

    ◦ enhance core strength and overall body composition.

3. Bench Press:

    ◦ stimulates upper body muscle growth, supporting testosterone levels, and

    ◦ improves chest, shoulder, and arm strength.

4. High-Intensity Interval Training (HIIT):

    ◦ boosts testosterone and growth hormone production, and

    ◦ improves insulin sensitivity and metabolic health.

5. Sprints:

    ◦ increase testosterone and growth hormone levels, and

    ◦ enhance cardiovascular health and fat burning.

6. Pull-ups/Chin-ups:

    ◦ stimulate upper body muscle growth, supporting testosterone production, and

    ◦ improve back and arm strength.

7. Kettlebell Swings:

- engage multiple muscle groups, promoting hormone balance, and
- improve cardiovascular health and core strength.

8. Resistance Band Exercises:
    - provide consistent tension, promoting muscle growth and hormone production, and
    - are versatile for full-body workouts.

9. Yoga or Pilates:
    - reduces cortisol levels, improving overall hormone balance, and
    - enhances flexibility, core strength, and stress management.

10. Farmer's Walks:
    - improve grip strength and overall body stability, and
    - stimulate growth hormone and testosterone production.

When performing these exercises:
- focus on compound movements that engage multiple muscle groups,
- aim for moderate to heavy weights with proper form,
- include both anaerobic (strength training) and aerobic exer-

cises,

- allow adequate rest between workouts for recovery and hormone optimization,

- stay consistent with your exercise routine.

Hormone health is also influenced by factors like diet, sleep, and stress management. Combining these exercises with a balanced lifestyle can help optimize hormone levels and overall health for men. It's always advisable to consult with a healthcare professional or certified fitness trainer before starting a new exercise regimen, especially if you have any pre-existing health conditions.

Hormones (and the potential for a relative lack thereof) play an integral role in the overall changes we associate with aging, whether that's because they affect how we feel day to day or because of the underlying risks for developing diseases. Take steps now to prioritize your diet, physical activity, sleep, and mental health, and you'll reap the benefits for years to come.

Hormonal Health Hotline: Your Top Ten Questions Answered

In this Q&A section, we're pulling back the curtain on male hormonal health, addressing everything from the impact of lifestyle choices to the realities of aging and hormone therapy, tackling the burning questions that men often ponder but may hesitate to ask. Navigating the world of hormones can feel like deciphering a complex code, but understanding your body's chemical messengers is crucial for overall health and well-being. Whether you're a young adult just starting to think about hormonal health or a seasoned gentleman looking to maintain your vitality, these answers will provide valuable insights.

I've compiled the top ten most frequently asked questions about male hormonal health, based on common concerns and curiosities expressed by men of all ages. Our goal is to demystify hormonal health, empower you with knowledge, and encourage proactive health management. Let's dive into these questions and unravel the mysteries of male hormones together. Remember, while this information is a great starting point, it's always best to consult with a healthcare professional for personalized advice tailored to your unique health profile.

Q1: At what age should men start paying attention to their hormonal health?

A: It's never too early! While hormonal changes become more pronounced after thirty, men of all ages should be aware of their hormonal health. Lifestyle factors can affect hormones at any age, so it's wise to start good habits early.

Q2: Can stress really impact my testosterone levels?

A: Absolutely. Chronic stress elevates cortisol, which can suppress testosterone production. Managing stress through strategies such as exercise, meditation, and proper sleep is crucial for maintaining hormonal balance.

Q3: I've heard about "man-opause." Is that a real thing?

A: Yes, but it's more accurately called andropause. Unlike the rapid hormonal changes women experience in menopause, men undergo a gradual decrease in testosterone levels, typically starting in their thirties or forties.

Q4: Can diet affect my hormone levels?

A: Definitely! A balanced diet rich in lean proteins, healthy fats, and vegetables supports hormonal health. Excessive sugar and processed foods can disrupt hormonal balance. Some foods, like cruciferous vegetables, can help balance estrogen levels in men.

Q5: Is "low T" (low testosterone) inevitable as I age?

A: While testosterone naturally declines with age, significant drops aren't inevitable. Maintaining a healthy lifestyle, including getting regular exercise and eating a balanced diet, can help maintain healthy testosterone levels as you age.

Q6: How does sleep affect my hormones?

A: Significantly! Poor sleep can lower testosterone levels and increase stress hormones. Aim for seven-nine hours of quality sleep per night to support optimal hormonal balance.

Q7: Can being overweight affect my hormones?

A: Yes, excess body fat can convert testosterone to estrogen, leading to hormonal imbalances. Maintaining a healthy weight through diet and exercise is crucial for hormonal health.

Q8: Are there any supplements that can boost my testosterone naturally?

A: Some supplements like Vitamin D, zinc, and magnesium may support testosterone production if you're deficient. However, it's best to consult with a healthcare provider before starting any supplement regimen.

Q9: How do I know if I have a hormonal imbalance?

A: Common signs include fatigue, decreased libido, mood changes, difficulty building muscle, and unexplained weight gain. If you're experiencing these symptoms, it's worth discussing with your doctor.

Q10: Is hormone replacement therapy safe for men?

A: When prescribed and monitored by a healthcare professional, hormone replacement therapy can be safe and effective for some men. However, it's not suitable for everyone and requires careful consideration of potential risks and benefits.

As we wrap up our "Hormonal Health Hotline" Q&A, and the book overall, it's clear that hormonal health is a complex and vital aspect of men's overall well-being. From the influence of lifestyle factors like diet, sleep, and stress, to the natural changes that come with aging, we've explored a range of topics that affect hormone balance. These questions and answers, along with the more detailed information contained in each of the chapters in this book, provide a solid foundation for understanding your body's hormonal landscape and recognizing when things might be out of balance. However, knowledge is just the first step. For some men, lifestyle changes and natural approaches may not be enough to address hormonal imbalances. This is where medical interventions can play a crucial role.

In our next section is a final overview of the various pharmaceutical options available for addressing hormonal imbalances in men. From testosterone replacement therapy to thyroid medications and beyond, the list of each treatment details how they work, their potential benefits, and important considerations to keep in mind. Understanding these medical options is essential for making informed decisions about your health. Whether you're currently considering hormone-related medications or simply want to be prepared for future conversations with your healthcare provider, this upcoming section will serve as a great referencing tool.

Chapter Eleven

Medications Used for Hormone Balance

Medications for Treating Low Testosterone
Testosterone Replacement Therapy

This involves supplementing testosterone levels through injections, gels, patches, or pellets. It's often prescribed for men with low testosterone levels (hypogonadism) caused by conditions like:

- injury or infection affecting the testicles,

- pituitary gland disorders,

- chemotherapy or radiation treatment, and

- genetic disorders like Klinefelter syndrome.

Specific drugs: testosterone cypionate (Depo-Testosterone), testosterone enanthate (Delatestryl), testosterone gel (AndroGel, Testim), testosterone patches (Androderm), testosterone pellets (Testopel).

How it works: directly supplements testosterone levels in the body.

Potential benefits: improved libido, increased muscle mass, enhanced mood and energy levels, better bone density.

Considerations: risk of acne, sleep apnea, enlarged prostate; regular monitoring required; may suppress natural testosterone production.

Human Chorionic Gonadotropin (hCG)

hCG is a hormone that helps stimulate the testicles to produce more testosterone. It can be used to treat low testosterone levels caused by pituitary gland issues or undescended testicles.

Specific drugs: Pregnyl, Novarel, Ovidrel.

How it works: stimulates the testicles to produce testosterone.

Potential benefits: can maintain fertility while treating low testosterone; may help with testicular atrophy.

Considerations: requires injections; risk of gynecomastia; may not be effective for all causes of low testosterone.

Clomiphene

This medication works by signaling the pituitary gland to release more hormones that stimulate testosterone production by the testicles. It's sometimes used as an alternative to testosterone replacement therapy.

Specific drug: Clomiphene citrate (Clomid).

How it works: stimulates the pituitary gland to produce hormones that boost testosterone production.

Potential benefits: can increase testosterone while maintaining fertility; oral medication.

Considerations: may not be as effective as direct testosterone supplementation; can cause visual disturbances.

Aromatase Inhibitors

These medications help prevent testosterone from being converted into estrogen. They may be used in combination with testosterone therapy to maintain proper testosterone-to-estrogen ratios.

Specific drugs: Anastrozole (Arimidex), letrozole (Femara), exemestane (Aromasin).

How it works: prevents conversion of testosterone to estrogen.

Potential benefits: can help maintain proper testosterone-to-estrogen ratio; useful in combination with TRT.

Considerations: risk of joint pain; may negatively impact bone density if used long-term.

Medications for Treating Erectile Dysfunction

There are several medications commonly used to treat erectile dysfunction (ED) in men. Here are some of the most common ones:

PDE5 Inhibitors

These are the most widely used medications for ED. They work by increasing blood flow to the penis, which helps achieve and maintain an erection. Some examples include:

- sildenafil (Viagra). This was the first oral medication approved for ED treatment.

- Tadalafil (Cialis). This medication has a longer duration of action than others in its class.

- Vardenafil (Levitra), and

- avanafil (Stendra).

How they work: increase blood flow to the penis by inhibiting the enzyme that breaks down cGMP.

Potential benefits: improved ability to achieve and maintain erections; increased sexual satisfaction.

Considerations: can cause headaches, flushing, nasal congestion; contraindicated with certain heart medications.

Alprostadil

This medication can be administered via injection into the penis or as a suppository inserted into the urethra (the tube that carries urine out of the body). It helps increase blood flow to the penis by relaxing the muscles and allowing more blood to flow in.

Specific drugs: Caverject, Edex (injections), MUSE (urethral suppository).

How it works: relaxes smooth muscles and increases blood flow to the penis.

Potential benefits: can be effective when oral medications fail; rapid onset of action.

Considerations: requires injection or urethral insertion; can cause pain or priapism (prolonged erection).

Thyroid Medications

Thyroid hormones play a crucial role in overall metabolism and can affect various aspects of men's health, including energy levels, weight, and sexual function. When the thyroid gland doesn't produce enough hormones (hypothyroidism), medication may be necessary.

Levothyroxine (T4)

This is the most commonly prescribed thyroid hormone replacement medication.

Specific drugs: Synthroid, Levoxyl, Tirosint.

How it works: Replaces or supplements the body's natural thyroid hormone (T4).

Potential benefits: Improved energy levels, better metabolism, enhanced mood, and potentially improved sexual function.

Considerations: May take several weeks to feel the full effects; requires regular blood tests to monitor dosage.

Liothyronine (T3)

Sometimes used in combination with T4 or alone in certain cases.

Specific drug: Cytomel.

How it works: Provides the active form of thyroid hormone (T3) that the body uses.

Potential benefits: May work faster than T4 alone; can be helpful for those who have difficulty converting T4 to T3.

Considerations: Shorter half-life, requiring more frequent dosing; may cause more side effects than T4 alone.

Natural Desiccated Thyroid (NDT)

Made from dried animal thyroid glands, usually from pigs.

Specific drugs: Armour Thyroid, Nature-Throid, WP Thyroid.

How it works: Provides both T4 and T3 hormones in a natural ratio.

Potential benefits: Some patients report feeling better on NDT compared to synthetic options.

Considerations: Not as standardized as synthetic options; may not be suitable for those with pork allergies.

Thyroid Hormone Receptor Agonists

Newer class of medications that can be used in certain thyroid conditions.

Specific drug: Tiratricol (TRIAC).

How it works: Activates thyroid hormone receptors without affecting thyroid hormone levels.

Potential benefits: May help in cases of thyroid hormone resistance.

Considerations: Not widely used; typically reserved for specific thyroid disorders.

Reviewing Your Options

In exploring the various medications available for treating hormonal imbalances and related conditions in men, it's clear to see that modern medicine offers a range of options to address these complex issues. From testosterone replacement therapy to medications for erectile dysfunction, these treatments can significantly improve quality of life for many men struggling with hormonal health concerns.

However, it's crucial to remember that medication is just one piece of the puzzle. The decision to start any hormone-related treatment should be made carefully, in consultation with a qualified healthcare provider, and after thorough testing and evaluation. These medications can have profound effects on the body and may carry risks as well as benefits.

Medication should often be viewed as a complement to, rather than a replacement for, lifestyle modifications. The foundations of hormonal health we've discussed throughout this book—including proper nutrition, regular exercise, stress management, and adequate sleep—remain fundamental to overall well-being and can often help minimize the need for pharmaceutical interventions.

Conclusion

Hormonal health has a tendency to take on a more prominent role in the discussion of women's health, partially because changes can be fairly abrupt. And while the term andropause—used to describe declining levels of testosterone in men—has intentional surface-level correlations with menopause, they are distinctly different processes. In men, the decline of testosterone over time occurs much more slowly. Due to the nature of a more subtle, drawn-out decline, the health effects are more easily attributed to general concerns or written off as simply "getting old."

Declining levels of hormones like testosterone are a natural part of aging. Some of these changes can feel inevitable, but you do have the ability to make a significant impact to promote a longer, more fulfilling, healthy life. This is true regardless of where you find yourself on your journey.

Recognizing those symptoms that can be associated with hormonal imbalance—like fatigue, changes in mood, or sexual dysfunction with low testosterone, or difficulty sleeping and tension with elevated cortisol—can help you gain a better understanding of the processes taking place in your body. This leads to more productive conversations with healthcare providers and a better understanding of how and why your personalized plan will likely benefit you.

Hormone replacement therapy can be very beneficial in some cases, but it's important to have a thorough discussion about its risks and benefits. In some instances, eating well, staying active, and sticking to healthy sleep habits may be all you need to stay on track and prevent broader health problems from developing. Starting small with healthier choices and setting practical, actionable goals can make a big impact.

In other cases, natural supplements can help bridge nutritional gaps or provide a helpful boost. Again, it's important to consider both the risks and benefits of natural supplements. In all cases, it's important to discuss significant changes in diet, exercise routines, and prescription or over-the-counter product use with a healthcare provider. This can help ensure your approach is not only safe but also effectively targets those areas that may be the most beneficial for you.

Aging and its associated hormonal changes are universal. Over the years, I've had the good fortune to lend support and guidance to many patients facing the same challenges. With every passing day we are all getting older.

What is also universal is the importance of knowledge. When you better understand the processes you are experiencing, the power is put back in your hands. Hormonal changes are no longer something that is simply happening *to* you; they are something that you can take positive action to manage.

I hope this book has served as a foundation to build upon. Our understanding of the human body, hormonal health, and strategies for improving our overall health is constantly improving. As you read this, studies are being conducted, and additional knowledge is on its way. Stay curious and keep exploring—there is always something more to learn!

Help Others Understand Their Hormones: Leave a Review!

Have you ever thought about how sharing your experience could help another guy out? Well, leaving a review for "Understanding Hormones for Men" is your chance to do just that! Your words could be the guiding light for someone else on their hormone journey.

Think of your review as planting a seed of knowledge. Your insights could grow into valuable advice for other men looking for answers about their hormonal health. Plus, it's a great way to look back on what you've learned and how it's changed your life.

Why does your review matter so much? Well, remember when you've checked reviews before buying something? Your honest thoughts could be that push someone needs to take control of their health. It's a small act that can make a big difference!

Here's where we need your help! If "Understanding Hormones for Men" has been helpful to you, please take a moment to share your thoughts. Don't worry, you don't need to write an essay - just be honest and speak from the heart. Here's how you can do it:

1. Go to the book's page on Amazon.

2. Find the "Write a Review" section Or Click Here!

3. Share what you loved about the book, what you learned, and how it helped you. (If you want to add a picture, that's awesome too!)

4. Hit submit and feel good knowing you've just helped someone else!

Here's a cool thought – imagine the ripple effect of your review. You're sharing something valuable, and that creates a wave of good vibes. Other readers will appreciate your help, and who knows, maybe someday someone will return the favor!

So, let's team up and make a difference. Share your thoughts on "Understanding Hormones for Men" and help other guys on their path to better health. Thanks for being part of this awesome community of men taking control of their hormonal health!

Thanks for your help!

Dr. Ashley Sullivan, PharmD

Ways to Connect:
Follow Dr. Ashley Sullivan, PharmD on Facebook, link below
https://www.facebook.com/profile.php?id=100092716005488

Website
https://ashleysullivanonline.com/

Join her FREE Facebook group "Compassionate Care and Holistic Advocacy with Dr. Ashley", link below.
https://www.facebook.com/groups/907620087038942

References

Akhgarjand, C., Asoudeh, F., Bagheri, A., Kalantar, Z., Vahabi, Z., Shab-Bidar, S., Rezvani, H., & Djafarian, K. (2022). Does Ashwagandha supplementation have a beneficial effect on the management of anxiety and stress? A systematic review and meta-analysis of randomized controlled trials. *Phytotherapy research: PTR, 36*(11), 4115–4124.

Alexander, E., Rutkow, L., Gudzune, K. A., Cohen, J. E., & McGinty, E. E. (2020). Healthiness of US Chain Restaurant Meals in 2017. *Journal of the Academy of Nutrition and Dietetics, 120*(8), 1359–1367.

Armstrong, L. E., & Johnson, E. C. (2018). Water Intake, Water Balance, and the Elusive Daily Water Requirement. *Nutrients, 10*(12), 1928.

AUA. (2018) Evaluation and Management of Testosterone Deficiency. *American Urological Association.*

https://www.auanet.org/guidelines-and-quality/guidelines/testosterone-deficiency-guideline Testosterone Deficiency Guideline - American Urological Association (auanet.org)

Banihani S. A. (2018). Ginger and Testosterone. *Biomolecules, 8*(4), 119.

Bhasin, S., Brito, J. P., Cunningham, G. R., Hayes, F. J., Hodis, H. N., Matsumoto, A. M., Snyder, P. J., Swerdloff, R. S., Wu, F. C., & Yialamas, M. A. (2018). Testosterone Therapy in Men With Hypogonadism: An Endocrine Society Clinical Practice Guideline. *The Journal of clinical endocrinology and metabolism*, *103*(5), 1715–1744.

Bremner, J. D., Moazzami, K., Wittbrodt, M. T., Nye, J. A., Lima, B. B., Gillespie, C. F., Rapaport, M. H., Pearce, B. D., Shah, A. J., & Vaccarino, V. (2020). Diet, Stress and Mental Health. *Nutrients*, *12*(8), 2428.

Campbell, M., Jialal I. (2022) Physiology, Endocrine Hormones. In *StatPearls*.

Chandrasekhar, K., Kapoor, J., & Anishetty, S. (2012). A prospective, randomized double-blind, placebo-controlled study of safety and efficacy of a high-concentration full-spectrum extract of ashwagandha root in reducing stress and anxiety in adults. *Indian journal of psychological medicine*, *34*(3), 255–262.

Chrubasik, J. E., Roufogalis, B. D., Wagner, H., & Chrubasik, S. (2007). A comprehensive review on the stinging nettle effect and efficacy profiles. Part II: urticae radix. *Phytomedicine : international journal of phytotherapy and phytopharmacology*, *14*(7-8), 568–579.

Cleveland Clinic. (2022). Here's the Deal With the Keto Diet and Type 2 Diabetes. *Cleveland Clinic Health Essentials*.

Corona, G., Sforza, A., & Maggi, M. (2017). Testosterone Replacement Therapy: Long-Term Safety and Efficacy. *The world journal of men's health*, *35*(2), 65–76.

de Bloom, J., Kompier, M., Geurts, S., de Weerth, C., Taris, T., & Sonnentag, S. (2009). Do we recover from vacation? Meta-analysis of vacation effects on health and well-being. *Journal of occupational health*, *51*(1), 13–25.

Duca, Y., Aversa, A., Condorelli, R. A., Calogero, A. E., & La Vignera, S. (2019). Substance Abuse and Male Hypogonadism. *Journal of clinical medicine, 8*(5), 732.

El-Sakka A. I. (2018). Dehydroepiandrosterone and Erectile Function: A Review. *The world journal of men's health, 36*(3), 183–191.

Fatemeh, G., Sajjad, M., Niloufar, R., Neda, S., Leila, S., & Khadijeh, M. (2022). Effect of melatonin supplementation on sleep quality: a systematic review and meta-analysis of randomized controlled trials. *Journal of neurology, 269*(1), 205–216.

Figueiredo, M. G., Gagliano-Jucá, T., & Basaria, S. (2022). Testosterone Therapy With Subcutaneous Injections: A Safe, Practical, and Reasonable Option. *The Journal of clinical endocrinology and metabolism, 107*(3), 614–626.

Finicelli, M., Di Salle, A., Galderisi, U., & Peluso, G. (2022). The Mediterranean Diet: An Update of the Clinical Trials. *Nutrients, 14*(14), 2956.

Gagliano-Jucá, T., & Basaria, S. (2019). Testosterone replacement therapy and cardiovascular risk. *Nature reviews. Cardiology, 16*(9), 555–574.

Hackney, A. C., Hosick, K. P., Myer, A., Rubin, D. A., & Battaglini, C. L. (2012). Testosterone responses to intensive interval versus steady-state endurance exercise. *Journal of endocrinological investigation, 35*(11), 947–950.

Hannou, S. A., Haslam, D. E., McKeown, N. M., & Herman, M. A. (2018). Fructose metabolism and metabolic disease. *The Journal of clinical investigation, 128*(2), 545–555.

Harvard Health Publishing. (2020). Is Testosterone Therapy Safe? Take a Breath Before You Take The Plunge. *Harvard Medical School.*

Hershner, S., & Shaikh, I. (2021). Healthy sleep habits. *Sleep Education.*

Hirotsu, C., Tufik, S., & Andersen, M. L. (2015). Interactions between sleep, stress, and metabolism: From physiological to pathological conditions. *Sleep science (Sao Paulo, Brazil)*, *8*(3), 143–152.

Hopper, S. I., Murray, S. L., Ferrara, L. R., & Singleton, J. K. (2019). Effectiveness of diaphragmatic breathing for reducing physiological and psychological stress in adults: a quantitative systematic review. *JBI database of systematic reviews and implementation reports*, *17*(9), 1855–1876.

HSPH. (2023). Shining the spotlight on Trans Fats. *Harvard School of Public Health*.

Hu, Nien-Chih MD; Chen, Jong-Dar MD; Cheng, Tsun-Jen MD, ScD. (2016). The Associations Between Long Working Hours, Physical Inactivity, and Burnout. *Journal of Occupational and Environmental Medicine*, 58(5):p 514-518.

Hu, T. Y., Chen, Y. C., Lin, P., Shih, C. K., Bai, C. H., Yuan, K. C., Lee, S. Y., & Chang, J. S. (2018). Testosterone-Associated Dietary Pattern Predicts Low Testosterone Levels and Hypogonadism. *Nutrients*, *10*(11), 1786.

Jones, M. E., Boon, W. C., Proietto, J., & Simpson, E. R. (2006). Of mice and men: the evolving phenotype of aromatase deficiency. *Trends in endocrinology and metabolism: TEM*, *17*(2), 55–64.

Koncz, A., Demetrovics, Z., & Takacs, Z. K. (2021). Meditation interventions efficiently reduce cortisol levels of at-risk samples: a meta-analysis. *Health psychology review*, *15*(1), 56–84.

Kotirum, S., Ismail, S. B., & Chaiyakunapruk, N. (2015). Efficacy of Tongkat Ali (Eurycoma longifolia) on erectile function improvement: systematic review and meta-analysis of randomized controlled trials. *Complementary therapies in medicine*, *23*(5), 693–698.

Kraemer, W. J., Häkkinen, K., Newton, R. U., Nindl, B. C., Volek, J. S., McCormick, M., Gotshalk, L. A., Gordon, S. E., Fleck, S. J.,

Campbell, W. W., Putukian, M., & Evans, W. J. (1999). Effects of heavy-resistance training on hormonal response patterns in younger vs. older men. *Journal of applied physiology (Bethesda, Md. : 1985)*, *87*(3), 982–992.

Leisegang, K., Finelli, R., Sikka, S. C., & Panner Selvam, M. K. (2022). *Eurycoma longifolia* (Jack) Improves Serum Total Testosterone in Men: A Systematic Review and Meta-Analysis of Clinical Trials. *Medicina (Kaunas, Lithuania)*, *58*(8), 1047.

Leitão, A. E., Vieira, M. C. S., Pelegrini, A., da Silva, E. L., & Guimarães, A. C. A. (2021). A 6-month, double-blind, placebo-controlled, randomized trial to evaluate the effect of Eurycoma longifolia (Tongkat Ali) and concurrent training on erectile function and testosterone levels in androgen deficiency of aging males (ADAM). *Maturitas*, *145*, 78–85.

Levy, B. R., Slade, M. D., Kunkel, S. R., & Kasl, S. V. (2002). Longevity increased by positive self-perceptions of aging. *Journal of personality and social psychology*, *83*(2), 261–270.

Ludwig, D. S., Aronne, L. J., Astrup, A., de Cabo, R., Cantley, L. C., Friedman, M. I., Heymsfield, S. B., Johnson, J. D., King, J. C., Krauss, R. M., Lieberman, D. E., Taubes, G., Volek, J. S., Westman, E. C., Willett, W. C., Yancy, W. S., & Ebbeling, C. B. (2021). The carbohydrate-insulin model: a physiological perspective on the obesity pandemic. *The American journal of clinical nutrition*, *114*(6), 1873–1885.

Martin, L. J., & Touaibia, M. (2020). Improvement of Testicular Steroidogenesis Using Flavonoids and Isoflavonoids for Prevention of Late-Onset Male Hypogonadism. *Antioxidants (Basel, Switzerland)*, *9*(3), 237.

Mayer, E. A., Nance, K., & Chen, S. (2022). The Gut-Brain Axis. *Annual review of medicine*, *73*, 439–453.

Mayo Clinic Staff (2022). *How much water do you need to stay healthy?*

Michnovicz, J. J., & Bradlow, H. L. (1991). Altered estrogen metabolism and excretion in humans following consumption of indole-3-carbinol. *Nutrition and cancer, 16*(1), 59–66.

Monson, N. R., Klair, N., Patel, U., Saxena, A., Patel, D., Ayesha, I. E., & Nath, T. S. (2023). Association Between Vitamin D Deficiency and Testosterone Levels in Adult Males: A Systematic Review. *Cureus, 15*(9), e45856.

Mulhall, J. P., Trost, L. W., Brannigan, R. E., Kurtz, E. G., Redmon, J. B., Chiles, K. A., Lightner, D. J., Miner, M. M., Murad, M. H., Nelson, C. J., Platz, E. A., Ramanathan, L. V., & Lewis, R. W. (2018). Evaluation and Management of Testosterone Deficiency: AUA Guideline. *The Journal of urology, 200*(2), 423–432.

Nassar, G. N., & Leslie, S. W. (2023). Physiology, Testosterone. In *StatPearls*.

Nenezic, N., Kostic, S., Strac, D. S., Grunauer, M., Nenezic, D., Radosavljevic, M., Jancic, J., & Samardzic, J. (2023). Dehydroepiandrosterone (DHEA): Pharmacological Effects and Potential Therapeutic Application. *Mini reviews in medicinal chemistry, 23*(8), 941–952.

NSF. (2022). Sleep by the numbers. *National Sleep Foundation*.

Pascoe, M. C., Thompson, D. R., Jenkins, Z. M., & Ski, C. F. (2017). Mindfulness mediates the physiological markers of stress: Systematic review and meta-analysis. *Journal of psychiatric research, 95*, 156–178.

Rachdaoui, N., & Sarkar, D. K. (2013). Effects of alcohol on the endocrine system. *Endocrinology and metabolism clinics of North America, 42*(3), 593–615.

Rahman, M. S., Hossain, K. S., Das, S., Kundu, S., Adegoke, E. O., Rahman, M. A., Hannan, M. A., Uddin, M. J., & Pang, G. (2021). Role of Insulin in Health and Disease: An Update. *International Journal of Molecular Sciences, 22*(12).

Rivas, A. M., Mulkey, Z., Lado-Abeal, J., & Yarbrough, S. (2014). Diagnosing and managing low serum testosterone. *Proceedings (Baylor University. Medical Center), 27*(4), 321-324.

Rubinow, K. B. (2017). Chapter 24: Estrogens and Body Weight Regulation in Men. *Advances in Experimental Medicine and Biology, 1043*, 285.

Russell, G., & Lightman, S. (2019). The human stress response. *Nature Reviews Endocrinology, 15*(9), 525-534.

Saleh, A. S. M., Wang, P., Wang, N., Yang, L., & Xiao, Z. (2019). Brown Rice Versus White Rice: Nutritional Quality, Potential Health Benefits, Development of Food Products, and Preservation Technologies. *Comprehensive reviews in food science and food safety, 18*(4), 1070–1096.

Sato, K., & Iemitsu, M. (2015). Exercise and sex steroid hormones in skeletal muscle. *The Journal of steroid biochemistry and molecular biology, 145*, 200–205.

Schulster, M., Bernie, A. M., & Ramasamy, R. (2016). The role of estradiol in male reproductive function. *Asian Journal of Andrology, 18*(3), 435-440.

Shahid, M. A., Ashraf, M. A., & Sharma, S. (2023). Physiology, Thyroid Hormone. In *StatPearls*.

Shin, B. C., Lee, M. S., Yang, E. J., Lim, H. S., & Ernst, E. (2010). Maca (L. meyenii) for improving sexual function: a systematic review. *BMC complementary and alternative medicine, 10*, 44.

Smith, S. J., Lopresti, A. L., Teo, S. Y. M., & Fairchild, T. J. (2021). Examining the Effects of Herbs on Testosterone Concentrations in

Men: A Systematic Review. *Advances in nutrition (Bethesda, Md.), 12*(3), 744-765.

Stress.org. (2022). What is stress? *American Institute of Stress.*

Swerdloff, R. S., Dudley, R. E., Page, S. T., Wang, C., & Salameh, W. A. (2017). Dihydrotestosterone: Biochemistry, Physiology, and Clinical Implications of Elevated Blood Levels. *Endocrine Reviews, 38*(3), 220-254.

Swithers S. E. (2013). Artificial sweeteners produce the counter-intuitive effect of inducing metabolic derangements. *Trends in endocrinology and metabolism: TEM, 24*(9), 431–441.

Tarkowská D. (2019). Plants are Capable of Synthesizing Animal Steroid Hormones. *Molecules (Basel, Switzerland), 24*(14), 2585.

Taylor, K., & Jones, E. B. (2022). Adult Dehydration. In *StatPearls*. StatPearls Publishing.

Thursby, E., & Juge, N. (2017). Introduction to the human gut microbiota. *The Biochemical journal, 474*(11), 1823–1836.

Timón Andrada, R., Maynar Mariño, M., Muñoz Marín, D., Olcina Camacho, G. J., Caballero, M. J., & Maynar Mariño, J. I. (2007). Variations in urine excretion of steroid hormones after an acute session and after a 4-week programme of strength training. *European journal of applied physiology, 99*(1), 65–71.

Travison, T. G., Araujo, A. B., O'Donnell, A. B., Kupelian, V., & McKinlay, J. B. (2007). A population-level decline in serum testosterone levels in American men. *The Journal of clinical endocrinology and metabolism, 92*(1), 196–202.

Tucker, J., Fischer, T., Upjohn, L., Mazzera, D., & Kumar, M. (2018). Unapproved Pharmaceutical Ingredients Included in Dietary Supplements Associated With US Food and Drug Administration Warnings. *JAMA network open, 1*(6), e183337.

Urology Care Foundation. (2023). Testosterone Therapy. *American Urological Association.*

Walter, K. N., Corwin, E. J., Ulbrecht, J., Demers, L. M., Bennett, J. M., Whetzel, C. A., & Klein, L. C. (2012). Elevated thyroid stimulating hormone is associated with elevated cortisol in healthy young men and women. *Thyroid research*, 5(1), 13.

Wang, Y., & Ashokan, K. (2021). Physical Exercise: An Overview of Benefits From Psychological Level to Genetics and Beyond. *Frontiers in Physiology.*

Watso, J. C., & Farquhar, W. B. (2019). Hydration Status and Cardiovascular Function. *Nutrients*, 11(8), 1866.

Whittaker, J., & Wu, K. (2021). Low-fat diets and testosterone in men: Systematic review and meta-analysis of intervention studies. *The Journal of steroid biochemistry and molecular biology*, 210, 105878.

Whitworth, J. A., Williamson, P. M., Mangos, G., & Kelly, J. J. (2005). Cardiovascular Consequences of Cortisol Excess. *Vascular Health and Risk Management*, 1(4), 291-299.

Wu, A., Shi, Z., Martin, S., Vincent, A., Heilbronn, L., & Wittert, G. (2018). Age-related changes in estradiol and longitudinal associations with fat mass in men. *PloS one*, 13(8), e0201912.

Xiong, X., Wu, Q., Zhang, L., Gao, S., Li, R., Han, L., Fan, M., Wang, M., Liu, L., Wang, X., Zhang, C., Xin, Y., Li, Z., Huang, C., & Yang, J. (2022). Chronic stress inhibits testosterone synthesis in Leydig cells through mitochondrial damage via Atp5a1. *Journal of Cellular and Molecular Medicine*, 26(2), 354-363.

Yanagi, S., Sato, T., Kangawa, K., & Nakazato, M. (2018) The Homeostatic Force of Ghrelin. *Cell Metabolism.*